Calcium Antagonism and
ATHEROSCLEROSIS

G V R Born MD DSc (hc) FRCP FRS

Director, The William Harvey Research Institu
St Bartholomew's Hospital Medical College
Charterhouse Square, London

D J Triggle PhD

Dean of the School of Pharmacy
Distinguished University Professor
State University of New York

P A Poole-Wilson MD FRCP

Professor of Cardiology
National Heart and Lung Institute, London

With compliments

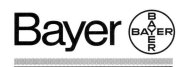

British Library Cataloguing in Publication data
Born, G.V.R.
     Calcium antagonism and atherosclerosis.
     I. Title II. Triggle, D.J.
     III. Poole-Wilson, P.A. (Philip Alexander)
     616.136

ISBN 1-870026-13-6

Project editor: John Dalton
Illustration: Maurizia Merati
Typesetting: Danielle Budd
Index: Doreen Blake
Printed in Hong Kong by Excel Printing

Front cover picture: An atheromatous plaque at the bifurcation
of a common carotid artery. The plaque shows patchy
calcification. By courtesy of N. Woolf, University College and
Middlesex School of Medicine, London, UK.

Contents

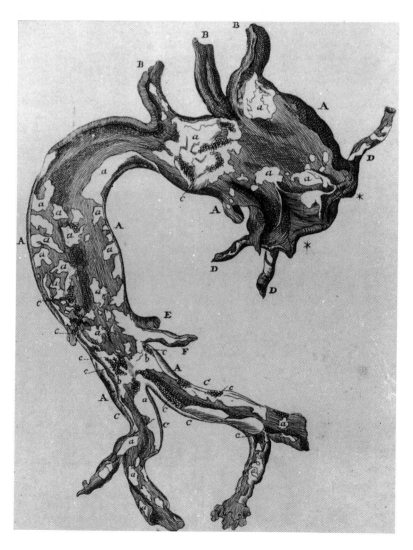

Fig. 1. The aorta of Johann Jakob Wepfer (deceased 1695). The above illustration appears in the posthumous edition of his *Observationes Medico-Practicae de Affectibus Capitis Internis et Externis* (1727).

1 Calcium and atherosclerosis

Introduction

Calcification as a feature of advanced atherosclerosis has been re-cognized *post mortem* for centuries. One of the first records of atherosclerotic calcification appears to be the illustration of the aorta of a famous physician, Johann Jakob Wepfer, who died at the age of 75 in 1695. The illustration opposite (Fig. 1) appeared in 1727 in the posthumous edition of his own *'Observationes Medico-Practicae de Affectibus Capitis Internis et Externis'*. The internal coat of the aorta is described as ruptured, lacerated and rotten, and to contain 'bone-hard', presumably calcified plaques. Because calcium, unlike lipids, is not present in obvious ways in earlier lesions as they appear in the postmortem room, it was generally assumed that calcium was not involved in the pathogenesis of the disease, and calcification was relegated to the role of one of several late, more or less terminal complications. This assumption has only lately been questioned, largely as a result of the work of A. Fleck-enstein and his co-workers. Our present knowledge of the origin and effects of calcium in atherosclerosis, and how this knowledge is affecting approaches to prevention and treatment, is the topic of this book.

To set the scene it is essential to give a brief, necessarily over-simplified account of the natural history of human atherosclerosis as it has been generally understood before the emergence of the calcium factor, which is then discussed in more detail. This should go a little way towards correcting 'the striking numerical discrep-ancy between the nearly uncountable publications concerned with disturbances in arterial lipid content and the few papers that refer to the patho-physiology of arterial calcium metabolism' [1].

The Cinderella status of the topic calcium in atherosclerosis is shown by two excellent recent books, one on arterial wall dis-eases in general [2] and the other on atheroma in particular [3], containing 684 and 114 pages, respectively. In each of these, the index contains a single page reference to calcium antagonists, and the text a single paragraph on calcification. This is not surprising in view of the fact that knowledge about the calcium contribution is still so limited.

The clinical impact of atherosclerosis

Atherosclerosis is the disease of arteries responsible for myocar-dial infarction and strokes, as well as for their respective precur-sor disorders angina pectoris and transient ischaemic attacks of the brain. This makes atherosclerosis the commonest cause of disabil-ity and death in the UK and in many other developed countries. The validity of this generalization has not been diminished by the decreasing incidence of coronary heart disease in the USA, where it has dropped by approximately 30% since the 1960s. The reasons for this downward trend remain obscure, but it is a hopeful indication that it is possible to arrest and reverse the increases in coronary heart disease that still afflict much of the world. In most countries the incidence remains high even when there are no increases (Fig. 2). The clinical epidemiology of atherosclerosis varies considerably between countries, depending on the prevalence of different risk factors. In the UK, mortality from atherosclerosis is predominantly due to coronary artery disease, which contributes to at least one-quarter of the total mortality in the country (Fig. 3).

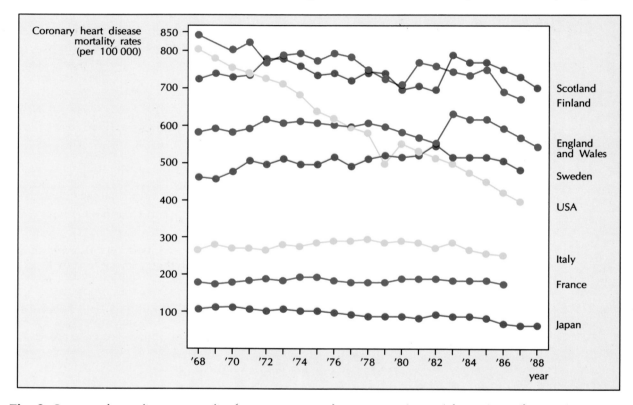

Fig. 2. Coronary heart disease mortality (rates per 100 000) in men aged 35–74 (age-adjusted). Data from the World Health Organization.

Population 56 million
660,000 die annually
177,000 from ischaemic heart disease
55,000 are under 70 years old
⅔ die outside hospital
½ die suddenly
40% of males dying aged 45–55 years

Fig. 3. Coronary artery disease – recent situation in the UK.

Atherosclerosis is an ancient disease. Arteries of Egyptian mummies dating from 1580 BC to AD 525 show typical plaques, so that the disease clearly occurred in ancient Egypt, at least amongst the mummified — presumably the upper classes. By the 18th and 19th centuries there were detailed descriptions of atherosclerosis in textbooks on morbid anatomy. It was Edward Jenner, famous for the discovery of vaccination, who in about 1771 first noted the relationship between coronary sclerosis and the symptoms of angina pectoris. In 1850 Cruveilhier described the association of arterial wall lesions with obstructive thrombosis inside the vessels. This was confirmed repeatedly throughout the following century and established as the dominant mechanism responsible for the common ischaemic diseases of the heart and the brain, myocardial infarction and stroke, respectively. The reason why the occurrence of these disorders is sudden and unpredictable was established comparatively recently with the demonstration that in the great majority of cases of fatal myocardial infarction the coronary thrombus has formed in relation to fresh fissures in atherosclerotic plaques [4–6]. Thus plaque fissuring is the initiating event; work now in progress is attempting to determine in what way fissuring may depend on the cellular and biochemical composition of plaques [7–9].

Plaque fissuring and thrombosis are terminal stages in the atherosclerotic disease process. Our understanding of the initial stages has been greatly advanced in this century through the study of animal models in which the pathogenesis is similar to that of humans and in which the progress of the disease is much more rapid (weeks and months) than it is in humans (years and decades). Elucidation of atherogenic mechanisms is using disciplines as diverse as epidemiology, genetics, molecular biology and fluid mechanics. Until recently these methodologies have been used predominantly for determining the roles of the lipid and cellular components of atheromatous lesions. Compared with these approaches, those intended to clarify the role of the calcium component are only at the beginning.

The lesions of atherosclerosis
Fatty streaks
When atherosclerotic arteries are examined *post mortem* in subjects of different ages it is evident that soft, yellowish lipid-rich lesions represent an earlier stage of the disease than hard, grey, fibrous and calcified plaques. The idea that lipids are a primary factor in the pathogenesis came initially from Rudolf von Virchow in 1862. He proposed that atheromatous lesions accumulate lipids from the blood plasma by 'insudation' into the arterial walls. Virchow's view on the origin of a lesion that impressed itself daily on pathologists in the postmortem room had the effect of concentrating research on the lipid aspect; since the first experimental demonstration by Anitschkow [10] that a cholesterol-rich diet produces arterial lesions in rabbits broadly similar to the early lesions in man, there has been spectacular progress with the elucidation of the role of lipids, particularly low-density lipoprotein (LDL), in atherogenesis [11,12].

Indeed, the first indication of the atherosclerotic abnormality is the presence of accumulations of lipid in the intima of susceptible arteries (Fig. 4). These initial lesions are known as 'fatty streaks' and have been classified by the World Health Organization (WHO) as stage I of atherosclerosis. In populations in which the disease is endemic, lipid lesions are commonly seen in young children at autopsy and even in aborted fetuses, showing that the atheromatous process can begin very early in life [13]. At first the lesions are small and separate, with characteristic patterns of distribution which will be discussed later. With increasing age the lesions enlarge, laterally within the intima so that neighbouring lesions merge, and outwards into the arterial lumen where they appear as raised, yellowish, soft plaques (Fig. 5). In cross-section the lesions usually appear as crescent-shaped encroachments into the lumen, in which a 'pool' of lipid material is covered by a fibrous 'cap', which in turn is covered by intact, apparently normal endothelium (Fig. 6). The lipid is predominantly the LDL of the plasma. The predominant cells in these fatty lesions are macrophages, which are derived from the monocytes of the blood [14,15].

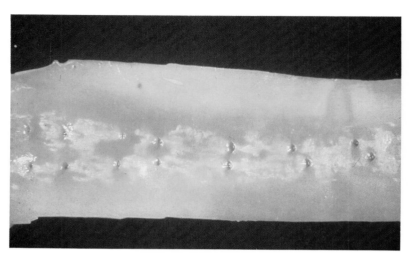

Fig. 4. Fatty streaks in human aorta. The aorta has been opened and pinned flat to allow examination of the intimal surface *en face*. On the intimal surface are elongated yellow areas barely raised above the surface; these are fatty streaks. There are also some smaller discrete focal depositions of lipid (fatty dot).

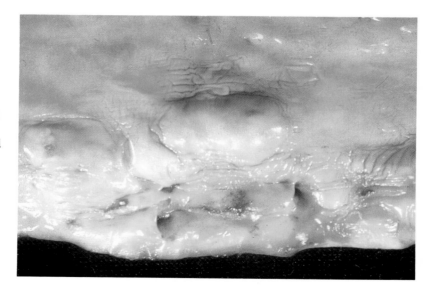

Fig. 5. Raised plaque in human aorta. The aorta has been opened to view the intimal surface *en face*. There is a large oval elevated lesion, the surface of which is yellow in some areas, white in others. The colour reflects different depths at which lipid lies within the plaque. The aorta also contains a smaller raised plaque and some fatty dots. By courtesy of M.J. Davies, St George's Hospital, London, UK.

In the proteoglycan-rich subendothelial spaces of the intima the macrophages avidly ingest LDL to turn into lipid-laden 'foam cells'. Considerable progress has been made with the elucidation of the processes by which LDL and macrophages pass through the endothelium and come together to produce the foam cells in the intima.

Fig. 6. (a) Diagrammatic representation of an atheromatous plaque in a medium sized artery such as the coronary in transverse section. The plaque is situated eccentrically with retention of a segment of normal vessel in which vasomotor tonal variation can occur. The plaque contains a pool of lipid separated from the lumen by a cap of intimal fibrous tissue. (b) Histological appearance of a human coronary plaque. The plaque contains a large clear central area in which lipid has been dissolved out during histological processing of the tissue. The base of the lipid pool at the junction with the media is deep purple in colour, indicative of calcification. By courtesy of M.J. Davies, St George's Hospital, London, UK.

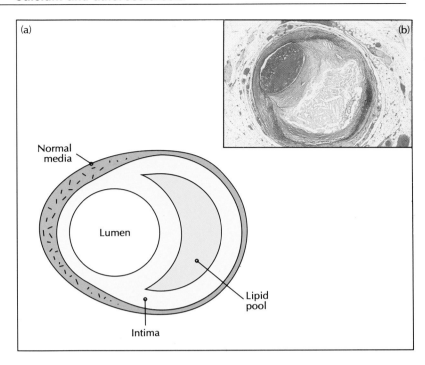

LDL uptake

Plasma LDL passes through arterial endothelium by transcytosis, apparently within the plasmalemmal vesicles that are characteristic of endothelial cells [16,17] and identical with the pinosomes in which lipoprotein particles were first demonstrated by autoradiography [18]. That LDL enters arterial walls by a mechanism that does not involve endothelial high-affinity receptors [19] is shown by the fact that the uptake of reductively methylated LDL that is not recognized by these receptors [20] is similar to that of native LDL [21]. It has been proposed that LDL is able to leak from the plasma into the intima in lesion-prone sites through endothelial gaps [22] that are associated with increased cell turnover at those sites [23]. However, there is contrary evidence in the demonstration that the clearance of plasma LDL is unchanged when wide interendothelial gaps are induced pharmacologically throughout a large part of the circulation [24]. Thus at present, it seems that the atherogenic passage of LDL into artery walls can be satisfactorily accounted for by transcytosis through normal, intact endothelium and that there is no necessity for postulating LDL leaking through gaps in the endothelium, whether physiological or pathological, as some form of 'endothelial injury' [25,26].

The predominant rate-determining factor of the arterial uptake of LDL is its concentration in the plasma. Although this can be shown experimentally [27], dramatic clinical evidence comes from patients with type II congenital hyperlipidaemia, in whom abnormally high LDL concentrations are associated with the occurrence of angina pectoris and myocardial infarction in adolescence or even in childhood [11,12]. Recent experiments with rabbits demonstrate that the atherogenic uptake of LDL is accelerated by adrenaline and noradrenaline at their pathophysiological plasma concentrations [28,29]. If this is also the case in humans, this finding would help to account for the increased risk of coronary heart disease in heavy smokers and others in whom there are increases in plasma catecholamines.

In its passage from plasma to arterial intima, LDL is in contact not only with endothelial cells but also with macrophages and smooth muscle cells in the subendothelial tissue. As a result of these contacts, LDL undergoes oxidative modifications [31]. The significance of this for atherogenesis is that it is oxidized LDL but not native LDL that is avidly taken up by macrophages [30,32]. The responsible receptor, the scavenger or Ac-LDL receptor, unlike the high-affinity B/E receptor, is not down-regulated by increasing intracellular cholesterol. This means that macrophages continue to internalize modified LDL until they become bloated with droplets of lipid [33].

Foam cell formation

Fatty streaks are characterized by large mononuclear cells full of lipid droplets. These are the classic 'foam cells' pathognomonic of atherosclerosis, and our understanding of their formation is now well advanced (Fig. 7). Foam cells are macrophages derived from the monocytes of the blood. Thus, the large numbers of foam cells in the lipid lesions are monocytes selectively transferred from blood to intima. This recruitment of monocytes begins with their adhesion to the endothelium. Significantly, the adhesion of these cells, like the transcytosis of LDL, is increased by hyperlipidaemia [14,34,35]. Adhering monocytes crawl through interendothelial junctions to reappear as macrophages in the subendothelial connective tissue. This directed migration is presumed to occur under the influence of specific chemoattractants. One of these, MSC-CF (McP-1), is a 14 kD monomeric cationic peptide [36] that is secreted by both smooth muscle and endothelial cells. Oxidized LDL is itself a chemoattractant for monocytes [37]. In the subendothelial space the monocytes undergo activation and differentiation into macrophages. During this process the cells increase in size and in metabolic activities [38]. In relation to atherogenesis, the most important of these is probably increased generation of superoxide ions that contribute crucially to the oxidative modification of LDL and thereby to the positive feedback resulting in foam cell formation.

To what extent other atherogenic lipoproteins, specifically very-low-density lipoprotein (VLDL) and lipoprotein (a) [Lp(a)], are taken up by macrophages via their scavenger receptor or by other mechanisms has still to be determined.

The lipid in mature fatty streaks is both intracellular in macrophages and smooth muscle cells and extracellular (Fig. 8), distributed between the fibrils and proteoglycans of the connective tissue and along the internal elastic lamina.

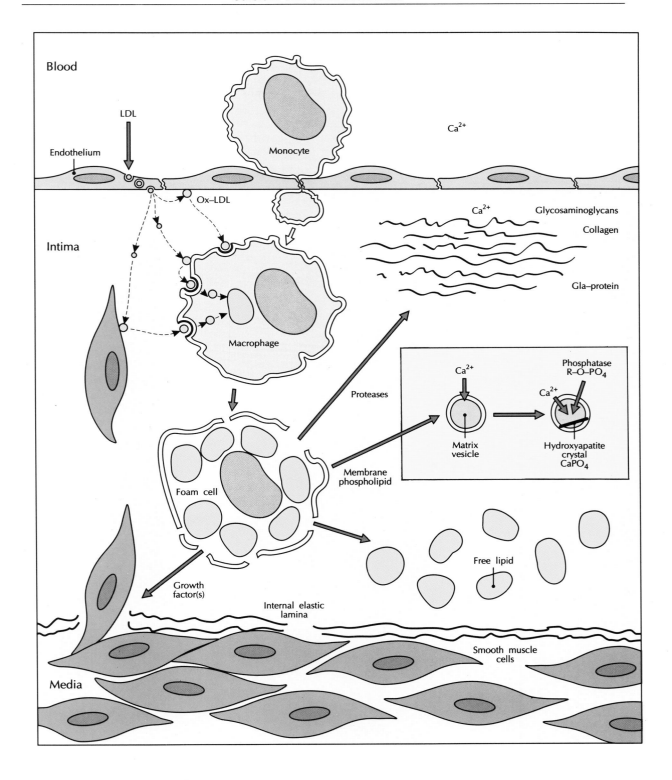

Fig. 7. Present evidence (simplified) of the contributions of low-density lipoprotein (LDL) and calcium (Ca^{2+}) to atherogenesis. For details see text.

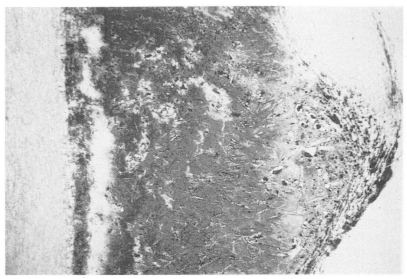

Fig. 8. General view of the centre of an atheromatous plaque, with the lipids deposited in the central zone of necrosis (staining red). In the region of the subendothelial fibrous cap (upper half of the picture) there are macrophages exhibiting extreme fatty degeneration. Published by permission (G. Assmann. *Lipid Metabolism and Atherosclerosis.* Stuttgart: Schattauer, 1982).

Fibrous plaque

Stage II lesions in the WHO classification are described as fibrous plaques. They are white rather than yellow and firmer than the lipid lesions. A pultaceous core consisting of cholesterol-rich lipid and collagen strands in variable proportion is covered by a fibrous cap of variable thickness (Fig. 9). Smooth muscle cells proliferate in the media and invade the intimal plaque, and new vasa vasorum are formed in the adventitia [39]. Although much remains to be explained about the pathogenesis of fibrous plaques, their derivation from preceding fatty streaks is supported by the fact that the arterial distribution of both lesions is similar and by the continuing presence of foam cells in fibrous plaques. Their uncontrolled overload with lipids, particularly with oxidized LDL, which is cytotoxic, [40] causes the cells to disintegrate.

Fig. 9. Two plaques in cross-section. In (a) the fibrous cap is thick (except at one end); in (b) the cap is very thin throughout. By courtesy of M.J. Davies, St George's Hospital, London, UK.

(a) 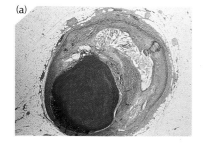 (b)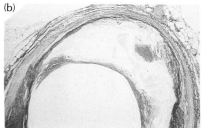

The released mixture of oxidized lipids and proteins comes to form the heterogeneous pigment known as ceroid, frequently described in human atherosclerosis [41,42]. Macrophages contain chemoattractants and growth factors, notably platelet-derived growth factor (PDGF), which are presumed to be also released from disintegrating foam cells and to be responsible for the migration and hyperplasia of medial smooth muscle cells in the intima [26].

Mature plaques

Plaques classified as stage III by WHO represent the final development in atherosclerosis. The plaques are bulky, stiff, and often complicated by necrosis, ulceration, haemorrhage and thrombosis. It is at this late stage that there is clear evidence of calcification (Fig. 10). Calcium deposits may occur in the superficial layer of the collagenous cap, in the intima below the plaque, and distributed around the extracellular lipid core (Fig. 11). Calcification visible on radiography indicates very advanced atherosclerosis (Fig. 12a, b).

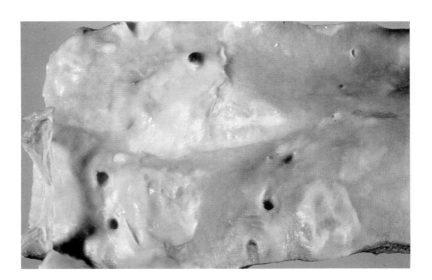

Fig. 10. Calcified aortic plaques. Several almost contiguous plaques with plate-like deposits of yellow-brown calcification on the surface.

There is evidence of an interesting difference in the composition of mature plaques in the aorta on the one hand and coronary arteries on the other. The atheromatous core of aortic plaques contains 30–65% lipids, based on dry weight, so that lipids make up a large proportion of the volume of the lesion [43]. In contrast, lipids contribute no more than 4–5% of the dry weight of coronary plaques whereas calcium salts make up almost one-half [44].

The most important question raised by calcification is whether and, if so, to what extent it contributes to the liability of mature plaques to develop fissures. This is because plaque fissuring is the initiating event in most cases of coronary thrombosis resulting in myocardial infarction [4–6]. Furthermore, repeated episodes of fissuring with thrombus formation underlie the clinical picture of unstable angina [45,46].

Plaque fissuring is obviously a complex problem, but it is clearly important to find out why it happens. As a starting point an anal-

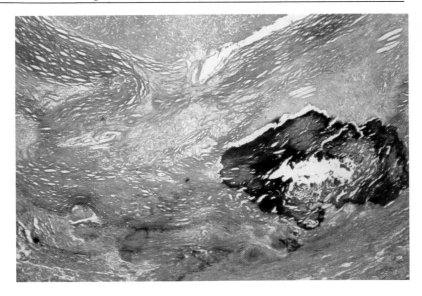

Fig. 11. Cross-section through a left anterior descending coronary artery. The lumen is on top and contains a recent, occluding thrombus. The fibrous cap of the arteriosclerotic plaque underneath, shown in red as acellular, dense, mostly collagenous tissue, is broken. Deeper in the plaque, on the right side of the microphotograph, is a focal calcification stained black. VanGieson–Elastin stain, original magnification (on Ektachrome slide) 40 ×. By courtesy of C.C. Haudenschild, Mallory Institute of Pathology, Boston, USA.

(a) 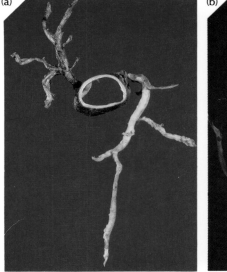 (b)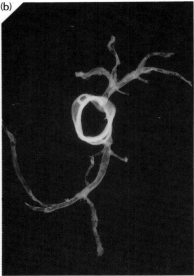

Fig. 12. (a) Aortic root and major coronary arteries dissected *post mortem* from the heart of a 60-year-old diabetic male smoker who died of myocardial infarction. Coronary arteriosclerosis is severe and diffuse, resulting in extreme stiffness and narrowing of all vessels shown. (b) Post mortem radiograph of specimen shown in (a), demonstrating advanced calcification of the arteriosclerotic lesions in these coronary arteries. By courtesy of C.C. Haudenschild, Mallory Institute of Pathology, Boston, USA.

ogy was suggested [47] between a fissuring plaque and the process of fatigue failure, the sudden appearance of a fault in metallic or plastic structures subjected to continuously variable forces over lengthy periods of time. Fatigue failure may be disastrous, for example, in the first jet aeroplanes, the Comets. The structural situation in an atheromatous artery is, of course, much more heterogeneous and complex, but there are similarities. The heart pumps blood through the coronaries, whereby their walls experience continuously variable stresses; it is conceivable that a minute weak point in a plaque might expand into a fissure, exactly as in fatigue failure. A computer model programmed to imitate the situation in an artery wall was adapted to introduce a small irregularity akin to an initial fault; this produced significantly increased stress at and around the irregularity [7]. As far as this goes it is compatible with the fatigue failure analogy.

The computer model has also shown that circumferential wall stress is maximal at the edge of a plaque cap over a lipid pool. This is also where about 50% of coronary fissures are found *post mortem*. Clearly, force distribution is just one of several determinants of fissuring.

Another determinant is mechanical resistance to breakage. Measurements of this have shown that the fracture stress of the centre of fissured plaques is lower than that of intact plaques, and this is associated with decreases in collagen and sulphated glycosaminoglycans. Therefore, deficiency or degradation of connective tissue matrix predisposes plaques with vulnerable configuration to fissure [48]. Fissured or ulcerated plaque caps contain significantly more macrophages than the caps of non-fissured plaques [9], suggesting a role for disintegrating macrophage-foam cells, presumably by releasing proteolytic enzymes, in the breakdown of connective tissue which predisposes plaques to fissuring.

The extent to which calcium is involved in the processes leading to plaque fissure is still unknown, specifically whether fissure is related to calcium content. Intuitively one would expect plaques with more calcium to be harder and more prone to the development of faults or cracks that are liable to progress to fissure; these questions remain to be answered.

Lesion distribution

After the atherogenic process itself the most important fact to be accounted for is the characteristic distribution of atheromatous lesions, both between and within arteries. The lesions, from the earliest fatty streaks to the fully developed, occur in some arteries, such as the aorta and coronary and carotid arteries, much more frequently and extensively than in others, such as the subclavian, brachial and mesenteric arteries [49]. Thus, the disease affects the largest arteries, rather than the middle-sized and smaller ones. The reason for this is not known, but may well be complex. A possible clue is the observation that in the frequently affected large arteries on the surface of the heart the lesions end abruptly as the vessels dip into the myocardium (Fig. 13a, b). By then the vessels are indeed somewhat smaller, but the contrast is very striking. In this particular situation an intriguing explanation would be the inability of LDL to accumulate in arteries that are continually being squeezed by the contractions of the heart.

Within a susceptible artery, lesions generally begin at and extend from branch orifices, for example at the origins of the intercostals from the aorta (Fig. 14), at the origin of the left anterior descending coronary artery, and at the carotid bifurcation. Although recognized early in this century [50], conclusive evidence had to await

Fig. 13. (a) Coronary artery on the surface of the myocardium showing typical advanced atheromatous lesion. (b) Similar-sized coronary artery without significant atheromatous changes where it is almost surrounded by myocardium. By courtesy of J. Wallwork, Papworth Hospital, Cambridge, UK.

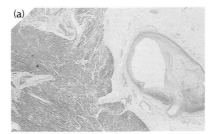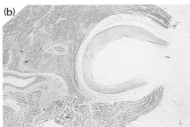

methods for mapping atheromatous lesions in major arteries [51]. For this purpose arteries are opened longitudinally and stained with lipid-soluble dyes such as Sudan IV, and the stained areas are evaluated in standardized arterial segments [52].

Fig. 14. Initial appearance of lipid lesions in the aorta of a young child. The aorta was stained with a fat-soluble dye which makes lipid deposits appear red. The deposits are at the orifices of the intercostal arteries.

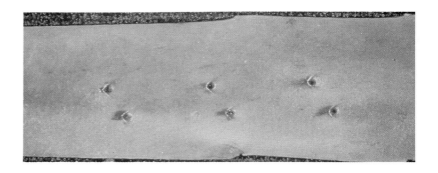

These techniques have been further developed to quantify the spatial distribution of stained lesions by computerized image analysis, providing 'probability-of-occurrence-maps' [53,54]. Such measurements have established the distribution patterns of atherosclerotic lesions in important arteries such as the major coronary arteries (Fig. 15) [55].

Two kinds of explanations have been proposed. One is based on evidence that the endothelium over lesion-prone areas is more permeable to macromolecules than elsewhere. Thus, lesion-prone areas are selectively stained by the azo dye Evans Blue when it is injected into the circulation. Evans Blue binds to plasma albumin so that blueing of the vessel wall indicates leakage of the dye–albumin complex [56,57]. Lesion-prone areas also accumulate fibrinogen [58] and LDL [59,60]. How the increase in permeability comes about is uncertain. The replacement rate of endothelial cells is greater at lesion-prone sites than elsewhere [23,61]; it has been suggested that temporary gaps that appear between dividing cells provide leakage paths for macromolecules. Alternatively, leakage may be favoured because the endothelial glycocalyx is exceptionally thin over those sites [34]. In pigs that develop atherosclerosis,

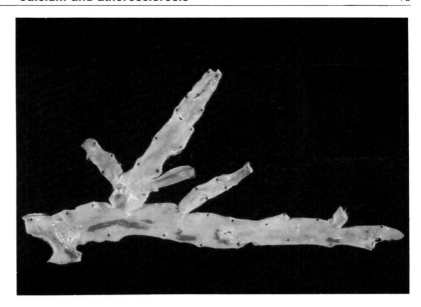

Fig. 15. Upstream region of fixed, stained left coronary artery demonstrating early fatty plaques (red staining areas). Published by permission [55].

whether spontaneously with ageing or more rapidly because of extra fat in the diet, the distribution of sudanophilic areas in the aorta is the same as that of areas stained by the Evans Blue technique [62,63].

Evidence of this kind has given rise to the proposition that the endothelium over lesion-prone sites favours the passage of LDL and other atherogenic macromolecules.

Another explanation is based on local haemodynamic factors. Lesion-prone areas are sited at arterial bifurcations and branchings where the blood flow, complicated enough in straight and unbranched segments of arteries, becomes even more complex because of vortex formation and flow separation into high and low shear fields. Evidence has therefore been sought for the presumption that the distribution of lesion-prone areas can be accounted for by haemodynamic effects. That *pressure* is involved is implied by the restriction of atherosclerosis to the large arteries in which the blood pressure is highest and by the fact that hypertension is a major risk factor for coronary heart disease. However, the mechanism whereby high blood pressure appears to promote atherosclerosis remains uncertain. The influence of *shear stress* has been subject to controversy. It had been proposed that lesions correspond to high shear [64,65], the link being 'endothelial injury' [66,67]. These notions have been disproved by quantitative analyses of the distribution of atherosclerotic lesions in coronary and carotid arteries [52,55]; these analyses have, on the contrary, established the association of atherosclerosis with low wall shear stress. The reason is not known, but may be related to the mass transport of atherogenic proteins between plasma and vessel wall [68].

In relation to the possible role of calcium in atherogenesis, an important question still to be answered is whether or not there are similarities between the distribution of lipids and of calcium, both between and within arteries.

The emergence of calcium

As pointed out earlier, until quite recently there was little consideration of the possibility that calcium, so obvious in late lesions, might be involved in the initial stages of atherosclerosis. Yet clues that this might indeed be so came from both human pathology and animal experiments. Thus, calcareous deposits associated with the earliest lipid lesions were seen in arteries of newborn infants and children [69], in one series in as many as one-third of those examined *post mortem* [70]. In 1913, Anitschkow in Russia first produced atheromatous lesions in cholesterol-fed rabbits. In the same year, Katase [71] in Japan first observed that arteries could be damaged by calcium: the injection of soluble calcium salts into rabbits and guinea-pigs caused disintegration of the internal elastic lamina in the vessel walls. This report remained almost unknown, and subsequent work was mostly concerned with arterial calcification induced by excess vitamin D_3 as a possible model of human atherosclerosis [72], but which also has some resemblance to Mönckeberg's sclerosis of the media.

That calcium might be a primary factor in atherogenesis has emerged comparatively recently, essentially as one of the consequences of the discovery of the calcium antagonists by Albrecht Fleckenstein [73]. With his wife, Gisa Fleckenstein-Grün, and their co-workers, they have pioneered the study of the role of calcium in the pathophysiology of arteries. The evidence is essentially as follows. First, the increase in calcium in normal arteries that accompanies ageing is markedly accelerated by major risk factors for coronary heart disease, that is, cigarette smoking, hypertension and diabetes [74]. Second, atherosclerotic lesions from early fatty streaks to mature fibrous plaques accumulate calcium in excess of the accumulation of lipid. Third, the calcium antagonist nifedipine, among others, reduces the development of atherosclerosis in cholesterol-fed rabbits [75, 76]. Fourth, controlled clinical trials have recently demonstrated that long-term administration of nifedipine to patients with early coronary heart disease significantly decreases the appearance of new coronary lesions, detectable by quantitative coronary angiography, when compared with patients on placebo [77]. The first two of these points will be considered in this chapter and the last two in Chapter 3.

Calcium in normal arteries

The basis for considering effects of ageing, coronary risk factors and disease on arterial calcium is its concentration and functions in normal arteries. Calcium is an essential component of the structure and functions of arteries, as of all other tissues. In humans, during the first decade of life the overall calcium concentration in the walls of large arteries is about $10\,\mu g/mg$ dry weight [44]; the values are similar in the young of other mammalian species. This concentration evidently represents an essential minimum for the structural and functional requirements of normal arteries, where the distribution of calcium between the extracellular and intracellular compartments is much as in other tissues. The functions and control of cellular calcium are discussed in Chapter 2.

Age-dependent increase in arterial calcium

That the soft arteries of the healthy young give way to hard arteries in the elderly was connected with calcium over 50 years ago when it was shown that arterial calcium increases with advancing age [78]. Recently this relationship has been re-determined comprehensively and also related to the effects of age on arterial cholesterol [1,44]. Specimens of normal human arteries were obtained at 144 autopsies, covering the entire life span from 1 to 90 years. Samples from the descending branch of the left coronary artery, the superior mesenteric artery and the aorta were analysed for calcium and magnesium by atomic absorption spectrophotometry. From the first to the ninth decade of life the absolute amounts of arterial calcium increased seven times in the coronary artery, 20 times in the mesenteric artery and almost 100 times in the aorta. Thus, in normal human arteries there is a progressive and continuous increase in calcium content from childhood to old age (Fig. 16). In contrast, arterial magnesium, which is a little higher than calcium in childhood, shows almost no increase with age; there is therefore something specific about the increasing calcium. The age-related accumulation of calcium in arteries is usefully referred to as arterial 'calcinosis', which distinguishes it from the arterial calcification associated with atherosclerosis.

Over the age of 60, calcium appears to increase in the aorta and mesenteric artery more than in coronary arteries. This curious discrepancy is, however, more apparent than real, because it can be explained by excess mortality in those over 60 years old with advanced *coronary* calcification. It seems that coronary 'high calcium carriers' are eliminated precipitously from the advanced age groups if the coronary calcium content exceeds the upper tolerable limit [79]. This epidemiological observation appears to be *prima facie* evidence that excess calcium in coronary arteries makes a significant contribution to cardiac mortality.

The age-associated rise in coronary artery calcium has been compared with concomitant rises in free and total cholesterol [44] (Fig. 17). Between the first and the ninth decade of life, calcium rises from about 0.4 to 4.1 mg/g dry weight, free cholesterol from 2.3 to 7.3 and total cholesterol from 4.6 to 17.8 mg/g. As normal human coronaries, therefore, contain more free and total cholesterol than calcium, it appears that 'the quantitative predominance of cholesterol over calcium is a significant criterion of healthy coronary arteries during the whole life span' [44].

Calcinosis, the age-related increase in arterial calcium, is not limited to humans but also occurs in rats, cattle, horses and dogs, in which calcium rises four- to fivefold during the life span of 13–16

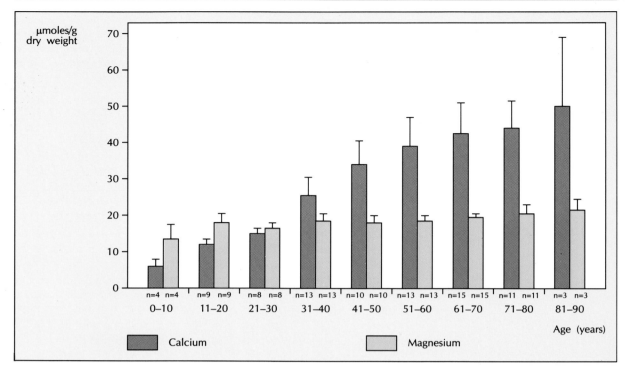

Fig. 16. Age-dependent increase of calcium in human coronary arteries. There is no similar increase in magnesium. Published by permission [74].

years [1]. This supports the conclusion that calcium accumulation is an inevitable, pseudo-physiological accompaniment of the ageing of the larger arteries, possibly having to do with the effect of the particular forces to which they are exposed on the retention of calcium within gradually changing wall tissues. However that may be, as none of these animals are subject to anything like human atherosclerosis, these findings would not support a pathogenetic link between the disease and the age-related calcium increase.

Acceleration of arterial calcium accumulation by coronary risk factors

In view of what has just been said, it is of great interest that several independent risk factors for coronary heart disease appear to accelerate arterial calcium accumulation [74]. The evidence [1] comes from histological and chemical analyses of arteries from 712 people. The vessels were obtained from healthy individuals (traffic or suicide victims or from amputations after accidents) and from patients with the major risk factors uncontrolled diabetes, hypertension, or excessive smoking. Compared with the normal age-related increase in arterial calcium, the process is significantly accelerated under the influence of these risk factors (Fig. 18): most in diabetics; somewhat less in heavy smokers; and somewhat less again in inadequately controlled hypertensives. It is not immediately obvious how these findings can be interpreted in the light of the conclusion from comparative studies that the age-related calcium increase bears no relation to the pathogenesis of atheroscle-

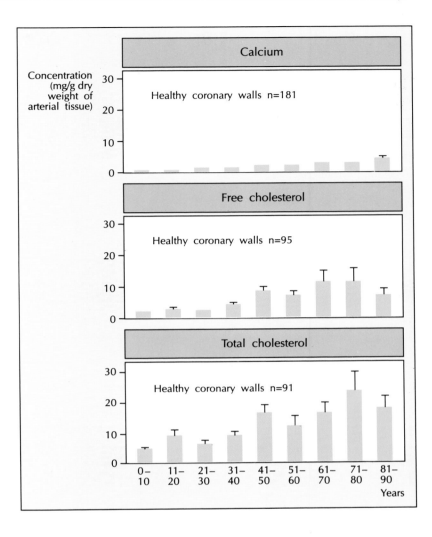

Fig. 17. Calcium and cholesterol in healthy human coronary arteries (age span 0–90 years). Published by permission [44].

rosis. It may be that the additional calcium measured under the influence of these risk factors is actually deposited not in the same way as the basic age-dependent calcium but in risk-factor induced lesions, so that the primary effect of the risk factors is to increase the number and sizes of plaques in which the excess calcium is located.

Calcium-binding constituents

In fatty streaks, the accumulating lipoproteins bring into the lesions the surface layers of acidic phospholipids; these appear to be the main extracellular calcium-binding molecules not present in normal intima up to the time when the lesion becomes dominated by monocyte-derived macrophages. As the macrophages turn into foam cells the internalized phospholipids presumably continue to be available for calcium binding. However, there appears to be no quantitative information about the association of calcium with lipids in this situation. The macrophages also bring with them the usual cellular complement of calcium-binding proteins; whether these can account for a significant proportion of the calcium present is uncertain.

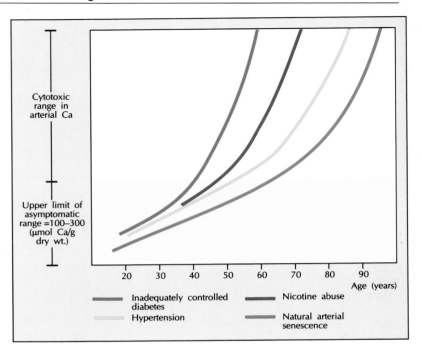

Fig. 18. Calcium overload of ageing arteries under the influence of risk factors. Estimations were made on the basis of observations in a total of 712 humans. Although there is considerable statistical variation in normal individuals, the arterial calcium accumulation, particularly in severe diabetics and excessive smokers undergoing leg amputation, is far beyond the physiological limits. Published by permission [1].

The progressive transformation of fatty streaks to fibrous plaques is associated with greatly increased amounts of calcium, as we have seen. The persistence of the lipid pool implies that the contribution of phospholipids to the total calcium-binding capacity is not greatly altered.

Increasing cellularity resulting from smooth muscle invasion presumably also contributes to a limited extent. Recent evidence establishes, however, that the predominant process responsible for calcium binding and deposition is cellular disintegration. This conclusion is based on the discovery that extracellular vesicles formed from the membranes of degenerating and disrupted cells become foci of calcium accumulation and calcification in a variety of tissues including bone [80]. Atherosclerotic plaques contain masses of these 'matrix vesicles' derived from the cell membranes of disintegrating macrophage–foam cells [81]. It is in these matrix vesicles that the first observable crystals of a calcium salt, calcium phosphate in the form of hydroxyapatite, can be seen electron-microscopically as electron-dense needles, lying against the inner surface of the vesicle membrane bilayer (Fig. 19) [80,82]. Thus calcification is initiated by the deposition of crystalline hydroxyapatite, a molecule with 10 calcium atoms, six phosphates and two hydroxyls in the unit cell [83]. Hydroxyapatite crystals, which are insoluble in body fluids at physiological pH, increase autocatalytically by homogeneous nucleation, the process in which initial crystals serve as nuclei or seeds for the formation of new crystals in the presence of physiological concentrations of calcium and phosphate in the extracellular fluid. Thus, calcification is initiated by the presence of ionic calcium in the fluid surrounding vesicle membranes (Fig. 20). Several membrane components that promote calcification have been identified [80]: (1) high concentrations of calcium-binding acidic phospholipids, particularly phosphatidyl serine; (2) high phosphatase activities (alkaline phosphatase, 5-AMPase, ATPase, inorganic pyrophosphatase and nucleoside triphosphate pyrophosphohydrolase) capable of producing local increases in inorganic phosphate; (3) complex proteolipids capable of nucleating hydroxyapatite, which have been isolated from calcified lesions in human and pig aortae [84]. The role of these proteolipids in atherosclerotic calcification has been made somewhat doubtful by their isolation from normal artery walls as well as from atherosclerotic lesions. However, proteolipids differ in both amino-acid and lipid composition [84]; thus their contribution to atherosclerotic calcification may turn on some particular biochemical property.

Fig. 19. Scheme for mineralization in matrix vesicles. During phase 1, intravesicular calcium concentration is increased by its affinity for lipids and calcium-binding proteins of the vesicle membrane and interior. Phosphatases (e.g. alkaline phosphatase, pyrophosphatase, or adenosine triphosphatase) at the vesicle membrane act upon ester phosphate of matrix or vesicle fluid to produce a local increase in PO_4 in the vicinity of the vesicle membrane. The intravesicular ionic product $[Ca^{2+}] \times [PO_4^{3-}]$ is thereby raised, resulting in initial deposition of $CaPO_4$ near the membrane. Published by permission (Anderson, *Metab Bone Dis Rel Res* 1978, **1**:83).

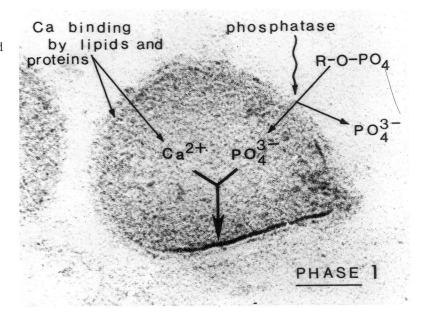

The evidence concerning calcification has recently been put together in the following hypothesis [80]. Matrix vesicles formed from disrupted foam cells attract extracellular calcium by the acidic phospholipids concentrated in the membranes. Phosphatases provide high phosphate concentrations. In the confined microenvironment of the vesicles the high concentrations of calcium and phosphate suffice to initiate deposition of calcium hydroxyapatite. The resulting crystals act as nuclei for progressive mineralization. With calcium and phosphate continuously available in the extracellular fluid, the autocatalytic, essentially physicochemical process proposed in this hypothesis could, in principle, allow calcification to proceed without limit, with disastrous effect on the organism. Although atherosclerotic calcification, once under way, does appear to progress locally, the lesions also contain controlling and limiting factors [80]. The deposition of calcium as the hydroxyapatite is antagonized by two components of connective tissue, proteoglycans and non-collagenous proteins with calcium-binding properties due to γ carboxy-glutamic acid (Gla) proteins. The presence of such proteins in calcified atherosclerotic tissue does not establish a role for them in the initiation of the calcification pro-

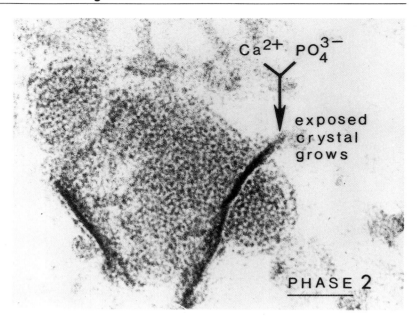

Fig. 20. With accumulation and growth, intravesicular crystals are exposed to the extravesicular environment. Phase 2 begins with exposure of preformed apatite crystals to extravesicular fluid, which in normal animals is supersaturated with respect to apatite, enabling further crystal proliferation. Matrix vesicles pictured are in rat growth plate cartilage. Published by permission (Anderson *Metab Bone Dis Rel Res* 1978, **1**:83).

cess [85]. On the contrary, it is possible that the presence of Gla proteins can be accounted for by their high calcium affinity following diffusional access from the circulating plasma, in which at least one non-coagulant Gla protein, the osteocalcin of bone, has been identified. The bone Gla protein known as osteonectin has the property of binding hydroxyapatite to collagen [86]. Whether there is a plaque protein with this function is unknown.

Effects of calcium accumulation

With the recognition that, on the one hand, arteries normally accumulate calcium throughout life and, on the other, that considerably more calcium is accumulated in the early lipid lesions of atherosclerosis, the view that calcification is merely one of several complications of advanced atherosclerosis has had to be revised. Instead, it seems likely that the age-related and the atheroma-related increases in calcium are distinct processes. To the extent that they occur separately, their effects on the properties and functions of arteries are presumably also distinct and can be considered separately. However, arteries affected by atherosclerosis are subject to both calcium-accumulating processes, so that the effects on function are certainly complex and incompletely understood.

Effects of calcinosis

The pseudo-physiological accumulation of calcium is only one of the changes in arterial walls associated with normal ageing [2]. Another change with ageing is thickening of the intima, mainly through increases in the connective tissue glycosaminoglycans and collagen. At the same time the internal elastic lamina becomes attenuated and tends to disintegrate, possibly under the influence of increased calcium as first demonstrated so long ago [71]. Incidentally, elastin may contribute to the stiffening of arteries with age through another mechanism [87]. Elastin has a high affinity for lipids including LDL [88], in the presence of which the access of hydrating water may be reduced. This may have an effect analogous to taking the elastin through its glass transition temperature, leading to increased stiffness of the elastin and so of the arterial walls in which it is embedded.

The functional effects of the thickening and hardening of arteries with increasing age are well known (Fig. 2 in [2]). Particularly important are the decreases in elasticity and distensibility, which are associated with increases in pulse wave velocity. The extent to which increased calcium *per se* contributes to these functional changes is not known.

Effects of calcification
It is worth recalling first that the location, growth and fate of plaques depend decisively on local haemodynamics. The development and distribution of calcification within any given plaque may also be strongly influenced by the haemodynamic environment. Conversely, this environment is affected by the position, size, shape and consistency of plaques. The site and extent of calcium deposits influence not only the plaques themselves but also the host arteries and the blood flow through them. These relationships are complex and still obscure. Little can, therefore, be done other than to give brief consideration to how calcification could affect plaque-related processes, that is, through progression, regression, and fissuring.

Plaque progression
There is both experimental and clinical evidence for the involvement of calcium in lesion progression. Thus, the development of atherosclerosis in rabbits on cholesterol-rich diet is retarded by several different calcium antagonists. The number of new coronary lesions quantified angiographically is significantly decreased in patients on nifedipine when compared with those on placebo, particularly in the early stages of coronary artery disease. Whatever the precise processes by which the drugs have produced these favourable results, they point to the conclusion that the formation of new lesions somehow depends on cellular calcium. These important findings are discussed in more detail in Chapters 2 and 3.

Plaque regression
Angiographically demonstrable regression of coronary lesions has been achieved in clinical trials by long-continued treatment with lipid-lowering drugs. Thus, the Cholesterol-Lowering Atherosclerosis Study [89] demonstrated significant regression as a result of treatment with colestipol and niacin for 2 years, and so provided a rational, mechanical explanation for benefits from cholesterol-lowering therapy. It was the first direct evidence for an effect of drug treatment on human atheromatous lesions.

This and another trial (see Chapter 3, page 54) have established the possibility of inducing lesions to regress; thereby they raise important questions. Could calcium antagonists, as well as decreasing new lesion formation, also induce regression of existing lesions? Could even early calcification impede or prevent regression produced by a lipid-lowering regimen, thereby diminishing this effect of lipid-lowering drugs? Could there be a calcification 'threshold', beyond which regression is no longer possible; and could it be this threshold which is influenced by calcium antagonists? And finally, could combined treatment with lipid-lowering and calcium blocking drugs bring about regression more effectively than either drug alone? These important questions await answers from appropriate clinical trials.

Plaque fissure

The cracking or rupturing of a coronary plaque is the immediate cause of arterial thrombosis which, if sufficiently obstructive, results in myocardial infarction or, if less obstructive and repeated, unstable angina. Current attempts to understand the underlying mechanism(s) have been described in an earlier section. As far as calcium is concerned, nothing quantitative is yet known about its contribution to plaque fracture mechanics, that is whether calcified plaques break more or less easily than non-calcified ones. In so far as calcification causes plaques to harden, their ability to move and to bend as a whole in response to the pulsatile blood pressure would be expected to decrease. Furthermore, calcification does not proceed uniformly but patchily so that haemodynamic forces impose internal shear stresses on plaques. It is reasonable to presume that these are major factors in determining the liability of plaques to crack, but the mechanical complexities have so far precluded analysis of plaque fissuring at this level. To a limited extent, the behaviour of plaques in their blood flow environment is now being analysed by the technique of ultrasound duplex scanning. This allows high-resolution imaging of plaques; assessment of plaque movement resulting from the cyclical stresses caused during each cardiac cycle; and the investigation of flow disturbances in their vicinity. One advantage of this technique is its ability to visualize plaque calcifications (Fig. 21) [90]. Correlations in sufficient numbers of plaque movements with calcification should provide information about its role in fissuring.

Conclusion

It is said that people are as old as their arteries. So the question is what ages one's arteries. Everyone knows from feeling the pulse that arteries are soft in the young and hard in the old, so that hardening is a sign of ageing. The mechanism responsible for arterial hardening presumably involves both fibrous thickening and calcium accumulation, though their relative contributions are uncertain. The calcium contribution is beginning to be properly established only through the comparatively recent work described in the foregoing sections.

That work indicates that there are two distinct processes responsible for the presence of arterial calcium in excess of functional

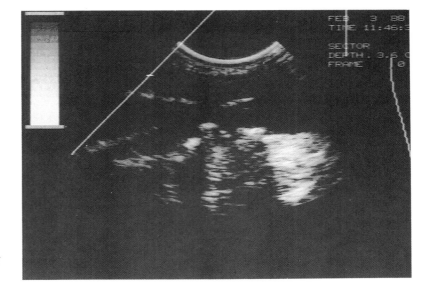

Fig. 21. Plaque at the origin of the internal carotid artery visualized by ultrasound duplex scanning. Areas of calcification present as high-level echoes producing shadows posteriorly. Less echogenic areas are also shown within the plaque which are consistent with intra-plaque haemorrhage. By courtesy of J.P. Woodcock, University Hospital of Wales, Cardiff, UK.

requirements. One process mediates the gradually progressive increase with increasing age in the calcium present in otherwise normal arteries with increasing age. This is apparently inevitable, occurs in other mammals, and can thus be thought of as pseudophysiological calcinosis. The mechanism of this process is not known. The other process, quite distinct from the first, is responsible for calcium deposition in atherosclerotic lesions that results in their calcification and is clearly pathological. On the facts so far known that appear relevant to this process, its essentials can be accounted for by the mechanism proposed by H.C. Anderson and associates (Fig. 19). It is presumably in this process that long-term treatment with calcium antagonists brings about the remarkable experimental and clinical effects which are fully discussed in the following chapters.

At the present time, knowledge of the role of lipids in atherosclerosis still greatly exceeds that of the role of calcium. So the position of calcium in atherosclerosis calls to mind the zoology student who came up to his final examination having concentrated on mammals and knowing nothing about insects. As bad luck would have it, he was asked about mosquitoes. Haltingly the student began: 'Mosquitoes are, ahem, nasty little buzzy things which, ahem, carry diseases. Mosquitoes, ahem, like to bite mammals. Now mammals are defined by the following characteristics . . . ' and away he went with his amassed knowledge. Students of atherosclerosis have concentrated on lipids when very little was known about calcium; that need be so no longer.

References

1. Fleckenstein A, Frey M, Zorn J, Fleckenstein-Grün G: Calcium, a neglected key factor in hypertension and arteriosclerosis. In *Hypertension: Pathophysiology, Diagnosis and Management* edited by Laragh JH, Brenner BM. New York: Raven Press, 1990: 471–509

2. Camilleri JP, Berry CL, Fiessinger JN, Bariety J (eds): *Diseases of the Arterial Wall.* Heidelberg: Springer, 1989.

3. Davies MJ, Woolf N: *Atheroma: Atherosclerosis in Ischaemic Heart Disease. 1. The Mechanisms.* London: Science Press, 1990.

4. Davies MJ, Thomas AC: Pathological basis and microanatomy of occlusive thrombus formation in human coronary arteries. In *Interactions between Platelets and Vessel Walls* edited by Born GVR,Vane JR. London: Royal Society, 1981: 9–12.

5. Davies MJ, Thomas AC: Thrombosis in acute coronary artery lesions in sudden ischaemic death. *N Engl J Med* 1984; 310: 1137–1140.

6. Falk E: Plaque rupture with severe pre-existing stenosis precipitating coronary thrombosis: characteristics of coronary atherosclerotic plaques underlying fatal occlusive thrombi. *Br Heart J* 1983; 50: 127–134.

7. Richardson PD, Davies MJ, Born GVR: Influence of plaque configuration and stress distribution on fissuring of coronary atherosclerotic plaques. *Lancet* 1989; ii:941–944.

8. Born GVR, Richardson PD: Mechanical properties of human athero-sclerotic lesions. In *Pathobiology of the Human Atherosclerotic Plaque* edited by Glagov S, Newman WP, Shaffer SA. New York: Springer, 1990.

9. Lendon CL, Davies MJ, Born GVR, Richardson PD: Arterial intima is locally weakened when macrophages are concentrated there. *Atherosclerosis* 1991: (in press).

10. Anitschkow N: Über die Veränderungen der Kaninchenaorta bei experimenteller Cholesterinsteatose. *Beitr Path Anat Allg Path* 1913; 56:379–398.

11. Goldstein JL, Brown MS: The low-density lipoprotein pathway and its relation to atherosclerosis. *Annu Rev Biochem* 1977; 46:897–930.

12. Brown MS, Goldstein JL: A receptor-mediated pathway for cholesterol homeostasis. *Science* 1986; 232:34–47.

13. Sinzinger H, Silberbauer K, Auerswald W: Quantitative investigations of indanophilic lesions around the aortic istia of human foetuses, newborn and children. *Blood Vessels* 1980; 17:44–52.

14. Joris I, Zand T, Nannari J, Krolikowski FJ, Majno G: Studies on the pathogenesis of atherosclerosis: adhesion and emigration of mononuclear cells in the aorta of hypercholesterolaemic rats. *Am J Pathol* 1983; 113:341–358.

15. Aquel N, Ball RY, Waldman H, Mitchinson MJ: Monocytic origin of foam cells in human atherosclerotic plaques. *Atherosclerosis* 1984; 53:265–271.

16. Vasile E, Simionescu M, Simionescu N: Visualization of the binding, endocytosis, and transcytosis of low-density lipoprotein in the arterial endothelium in situ. *J Cell Biol* 1983; 96:1677–1689.

17. Simionescu N, Vasile E, Lupu F, Popescu G, Simionescu M: Prelesional events in atherogenesis: accumulation of extracellular cholesterol-rich liposomes in the arterial intima and cardiac valves of the hyperlipidaemic rabbit. *Am J Pathol* 1986; 123:109–125.

18. Stein O, Stein Y, Eisenberg S: A radiographic study of the transport of I-labeled serum lipoproteins in rat aorta. *Cell Tissue Res* 1973; 138:223–232.

19. Vlodavsky I, Fielding PE, Fielding CJ, Gospadorowicz D: Role of contact inhibition in the regulation of receptor-mediated uptake of low density lipoprotein in cultured vascular endothelial cells. *Proc Natl Acad Sci USA* 1978; 75: 356–360.

20. Mahley RW, Weisgraber KH, Innerarity TL: Interaction of plasma lipoproteins containing apolipoproteins B and E with heparin and cell surface receptors. *Biochim Biophys Acta* 1979; 575:81–91.

21. Wiklund O, Carew TE, Steinberg D: Role of the low density lipoprotein receptor in penetration of low density lipoprotein into rabbit aortic wall. *Arteriosclerosis* 1985; 5:135–141.

22. Lin S-J, Jan KM, Weinbaum S, Chien S: Transendothelial transport of low density lipoprotein in association with cell mitosis in rat aorta. *Arteriosclerosis* 1989; 9: 230–236.

23. Payling-Wright HP, Born GVR: Possible effect of blood flow on the turnover rate of vascular endothelial cells. In *Theoretical and Clinical Haemorheology* edited by Hartert HH, Copley AL. Heidelberg: Springer, 1971: 220–226.

24. Born GVR, Shafi S: Evidence against the atherogenic passage of low density lipoproteins between vascular endothelial cells in conscious rabbits. *J Physiol (Lond)* 1989; 418:80.

25. Ross R: Atherosclerosis: a problem of the biology of arterial wall cells and their interactions with blood components. *Arteriosclerosis* 1981; 1:293–311.

26. Ross R: The pathogenesis of atherosclerosis – an update. *N Engl J Med* 1986; 314:488–499.

27. Van Hinsbergh *et al.*: *In vivo* and *in vitro* catabolism of native and biogically modified LDL. *FEBS Lett* 1984; 171:149–153.

28. Shafi S, Cusack NJ, Born GVR: Increased uptake of methylated low density lipoprotein induced by noradrenaline in carotid arteries of anaesthetised rabbits. *Proc R Soc Lond [B]* 1989; 235: 289–293.

29. Cardona, Born GVR: (in preparation).

30. Steinbrecher UP, Parthasarathy S, Leake DS, Witztum JL, Steinberg D: Modification of low density lipoprotein by endothelial cells involves lipid peroxidation and degradation of low density lipoprotein phospholipid. *Proc Natl Acad Sci USA* 1984; 81:3883–3887.

31. Morel DW, Di Corleto PE, Chisolm GM: Endothelial and smooth muscle cells alter low density lipoprotein in vitro by free radical oxidation. *Arteriosclerosis* 1984; 4:357–364.

32. Steinberg D, Parthasarathy S, Carew T, Chou JC, Witztum DL: Beyond cholesterol: modification of low-density lipoprotein that increases its atherogenicity. *N Engl J Med* 1989; 320:912–924

33. Brown MS, Goldstein SL: Lipoprotein metabolism in the macrophage: implications for cholesterol deposition in atherosclerosis. *Annu Rev Biochem* 1983; 52: 223–261.

34. Gerrity RG, Naito HK, Richardson M, Schwartz CJ: Dietary induced atherogenesis in swine. I. Morphology of the intima in prelesion stages. *Am J Pathol* 1979; 95: 775–792.

35. Gerrity RG: The role of the monocyte in atherogenesis. I. Transition of blood-borne monocytes into foam cells in fatty lesions. *Am J Pathol* 1981; 103:181–190.

36. Valente AJ, Graves DT, Vialle-Valentin CE, Delgado R, Schwartz CJ: Purification of a monocyte chemotactic factor (SMC-CF) secreted by non-human primate vascular smooth muscle cells in culture. *Biochemistry* 1988; 27:4162–4168.

37. Quinn MT, Parthasarathy S, Fong LG, Steinberg D: Oxidatively modified low density lipoprotein: a potential role in recruitment and retention of monocytes/macrophages in atherogenesis. *Proc Natl Acad Sci USA* 1987; 84:2995–2998.

38. Schwartz CJ, Valente AJ, Sprague EA, Kelley JL, Nerem RM: The pathogenesis of atherosclerosis: an overview. *Clin Cardiol* 1991; 14:1–16.

39. Barger AC, Beeuwkes R III, Lainey LL, *et al.*: Hypothesis: Vasa vasorum and neovascularization of human coronary arteries. A possible role in the patho-physiology of atherosclerosis. *N Engl J Med* 1984; 310:175–177.

40. Cathcart MK, Morel DW, Chisolm GM: Monocytes and neutrophils oxidise low density lipoprotein making it cytotoxic. *J Leukoc Biol* 1985; 83:341–350.

41. Pappenheimer AM, Victor J: Ceroid pigment in human tissues. *Am J Pathol* 1946; 22:395–413.

42. Porta E, Hartroft WS: In *Pigments in Pathology* edited by Wolnan M. New York: Academic Press, 1969: 191–235.

43. Small DM: Progression and regression of atherosclerotic lesions. Insights from lipid physical biochemistry. *Arteriosclerosis* 1988; 8:103–129.

44. Fleckenstein A, Frey M, Thimm F, Fleckenstein-Grün G: Excessive mural calcium overload. A predominant causal factor in the development of stenosing coronary plaques in humans. *Cardiovasc Drugs Ther* 1990 4:1005–1014.

45. Levin DC, Fallon JT: Significance of the angiographic morphology of localised

coronary stenoses. Histopathological correlates. *Circulation* 1982; 66:316–320.

46. Falk E: Unstable angina with fatal outcome: dynamic coronary thrombosis leading to infarction and/or sudden death. *Circulation* 1985; 71:699–708.

47. Born GVR: Arterial thrombosis and its prevention. In *Cardiology* edited by Haydase S, Murao S. Amsterdam: Excerpta Medica, 1979: 81–91.

48. Burleigh MC, Briggs AD, Lendon CL, Davies MJ, Born GVR, Richardson PD: Biochemical composition and fracture mechanics of cap tissue in human ulcerated and non-ulcerated atherosclerotic plaques. *Atherosclerosis* (in press).

49. Woolf N: *The Pathology of Atherosclerosis.* London: Butterworth, 1982.

50. Chiari, H: Über das Verhalten des Teilungswinkels der Carotis Communis bei der Endarteritis Chronica Deformaus. *Verh Dtsch Ges Pathol* 1905; 9:326.

51. Schwartz CJ, Mitchell JRA: Observations on localisation of arterial plaques. *Circ Res* 1962; 11:63–66.

52. Grottum P, Svindland A, Walloe L: Localisation of atherosclerotic lesions in the bifurcation of the main left coronary artery. *Atherosclerosis* 1983; 47:55–62.

53. Cornhill JF, Barrett WA, Herderick EE, Mahley RW, Fry DL: Topographic study of melanophilic lesions in cholesterol-fed minipigs by image analysis. *Arteriosclerosis* 1985; 5:415–426.

54. Cornhill JF, Henderick EE, Stary HC: Topography of human aortic sudanophilic lesions. In *Blood Flow in Larger Arteries: Applications to Atherogenesis and Clinical Medicine* edited by Liepsch DW. Basel: Karger 1990, 15:13–19.

55. Fox B, Seed WA: Location of early atheroma in the human coronary arteries. *J Biomech Eng* 1981; 103:208–212.

56. Packham MA, Rowsell HC, Jorgensen L, Mustard JF: Localised protein accumulation in the wall of aorta. *Exp Mol Pathol* 1967; 7:214–232.

57. Bell FP, Adamson I, Schwartz CJ: Aortic endothelial permeability to albumen: focal and regional patterns of uptake and transmural distribution of ^{125}I-albumin in the young pig. *Exp Mol Pathol* 1974; 20:57–58.

58. Bell FP, Gallus AS, Schwartz CJ: Focal and regional patterns of uptake and the transmural distribution of ^{125}I-fibrinogen in the pig aorta in vivo. *Exp Mol Pathol* 1974; 20:281.

59. Hoff HF, Bond MG: Apolipoprotein B localization in coronary atherosclerotic plaques from cynomolgus monkeys. *Artery* 1983; 12: 104–116.

60. Feldman DL, Hoff HF, Gerrity RG: Immunohistochemical localization of apoprotein B in aortas from hyperlipemic swine. *Arch Pathol Lab Med* 1984; 108: 817–821.

61. Caplan BA, Schwartz CJ: Increased endothelial cell turnover in areas of in vivo Evans Blue uptake in the young pig aorta.

I. Quantitative light microscopic findings. *Exp Mol Pathol* 1974; 21: 102–117.

62. Day AJ, Bell FP, Schwartz CJ: Lipid metabolism in focal areas of normal-fed and cholesterol-fed pig aorta. *Exp Mol Pathol* 1979; 21:179–193.

63. Bell FP, Day AJ, Gent M, Schwartz CJ: Differing patterns of cholesterol accumulation and ^{3}H-cholesterol influx in areas of the cholesterol-fed pig aorta identified by Evans Blue dye. *Exp Mol Pathol* 1975; 22:366–375.

64. Fry DL: Localizing factors in arteriosclerosis. In *Atherosclerosis and Coronary Heart Disease* edited by Likoff W, Segal BL, Insull W, Moyer JA. New York: Grune and Stratten, 1972: 40–104.

65. Fry DL: Hemodynamic forces in atherogenesis. In *Cerebrovascular Diseases* edited by Scheinberg P. New York: Raven Press 1976; 77–95.

66. Moore S: Injury mechanisms in atherogenesis. In *Vascular Injury and Atherosclerosis* edited by Moore S. New York: Marcel Dekker, 1981; 131–148.

67. Mustard JF, Packham MA: The role of blood and platelets in atherosclerosis and the complications of atherosclerosis. *Thromb Diath Haemorh* 1975; 33:444–456.

68. Caro CG: Atheroma and arterial wall shear. Observation, correlation and proposal of a shear-dependent mass-transfer mechanism for atherogenesis. *Proc R Soc London [B]* 1971; 177: 109–159.

69. Meyer WW, Lind J: Calcification of iliac arteries in newborns and infants. *Arch Dis Child* 1972; 47:364–372.

70. Helletzgruber M, Sinzinger H, Feigl W, Holzner JH. Initial arterial lesions – starting in foetuses? *Folia Anat Jugosl* 1975; 4:83–86.

71. Katase A: Experimentelle Verkalkung am gesunden Tiere. *Beiträge Path Anat Allg Path* 1913; 57:516–550.

72. Yogamundi Moon J: Factors affecting arterial calcification associated with atherosclerosis: a review. *Atherosclerosis* 1972; 16:119–126.

73. Fleckenstein A: History of calcium antagonists. In *Calcium Channel Blocking Drugs: Novel Intervention for the Treatment of Cardiac Disease. Circ Res* 1983; 52 (suppl 1):3–16.

74. Fleckenstein A, Frey M, Fleckenstein-Grün G: Antihypertensive and arterial anticalcinotic effects of calcium antagonists. *Am J Cardiol* 1986; 57: 1D–10D.

75. Henry PD, Bentley K: Suppression of atherosclerosis in cholesterol-fed rabbits with nifedipine. *J Clin Invest* 1981; 68: 1366–1369.

76. Watanabe N, Ischikawa Y, Mukodani J, *et al:* Nifedipine suppresses arteriosclerosis in cholesterol-fed rabbits but not in WHHL-rabbits. *Circulation* 1985; 72:111–281.

77. Lichtlen PR, Hugenholtz PG, Rafflenbeul W, Hecker H, Jost S, Nikutta P, Deckers JW: Retardation of coronary artery

disease in humans by the calcium-channel blocker nifedipine: results of the INTACT study (International Nifedipine Trial on Antiatherosclerotic Therapy). *Cardiovasc Drugs Ther* 1990; 4:1047–1068.

78. Bürger M: Die chemischen Altersveränderungen an Gefässen. *Z Neurol Psychol* 1939; 167:273–280.

79. Fleckenstein A, Frey M, von Witzleben H: Vascular calcium overload – a pathogenetic factor in arteriosclerosis and its neutralisation by calcium antagonists. In *New Therapy of Ischaemic Heart Disease and Hypertension* edited by Kaltenbach N, Neufeld HN. Amsterdam: Excerpta Medica, 1983; 36–52.

80. Anderson HC, McGregor DH, Tanimura A: Mechanisms of calcification in atherosclerosis. In *Pathobiology of the Human Atherosclerotic Plaque* edited by Glagov S, Newman WP, Schaffer SA. New York: Springer 1990: 235–249.

81. Tanmura A, McGregor DH, Anderson HC: Matrix vesicles in atherosclerotic calcification. *Proc Soc Exp Biol Med* 1983; 172:173–177.

82. Bonucci E: Fine structure and histochemistry of calcifying globules in epiphyseal cartilage. *Z Zellforsch* 1970; 103:192–217.

83. Posner AS: Crystal chemistry of bone mineral. *Physiol Rev* 1969; 49:760–792.

84. Romeo R, Augustyn JM, Mandel G, Daond AS: Characterization of nucleating proteolipids from calcified and non-calcified atherosclerotic lesions. In *Pathobiology of the Human Atherosclerotic Plaque* edited by Glagov S, Newman WP, Schaffer SA. New York: Springer 1990: 251–262.

85. Keeley FW, Sitarz EE: Characterisation of proteins from the calcified matrix of atherosclerotic human aorta. *Atherosclerosis* 1983; 46:29–40.

86. Termine JD, Kleinman HK, Whitson WS, Conn KM, McGarvey ML, Martin GR: Osteonectin, a bone-specific protein linking mineral to collagen. *Cell* 1981; 26: 99–105.

87. Lillie MA, Gosline JM: The effects of hydration on the dynamic mechanical properties of elastin. In *Physical Network: Polymers and Gels* edited by Burchard W, Ross-Murphy SB. Amsterdam: Elsevier, 391–401: 1990.

88. Podet EJ, Shaffer DR, Gianturco SH, Bradley WA, Yang CY, Guyton JR: Interaction of low density lipoproteins with human aortic elastin. *Arteriosclerosis* 1991; 11:116–122.

89. Blankenhorn DH, Nessim SA, Johnson RD, Sanmarco ME, Azen SP, Cashin-Hemphill MD: Beneficial effects of combined colestipol-niacin therapy on coronary atherosclerosis and coronary venous bypass grafts. *JAMA* 1987; 257:3233–3240.

90. Woodcock JP: Characterisation of the atheromatous plaque in the carotid arteries. *Clin Phys Physiol Meas* 1989; 10:45–49.

2 Calcium channel antagonists: sites, control and mechanisms of action relevant to the atherosclerotic process

Introduction

Calcium is a cation critical to cellular control. This was first recognized by Sidney Ringer (1836–1910), an English physician and physiologist, who in 1883 described the critical role of calcium in the maintenance of cardiac contractility [1]. Calcium is a ubiquitous intracellular mediator coupling cellular receptors to cellular responses (Fig. 1). These physiological events give way to pathological events under conditions of unregulated calcium entry, mediating death and destruction subsequent to cellular insults and the loss of metabolic control (Fig. 2). Accordingly, pharmacological control of cellular calcium movements is of major therapeutic interest and has led to the development of agents, the calcium antagonists or calcium-channel blockers, that are effective in the first-line control of cardiovascular disorders, including angina

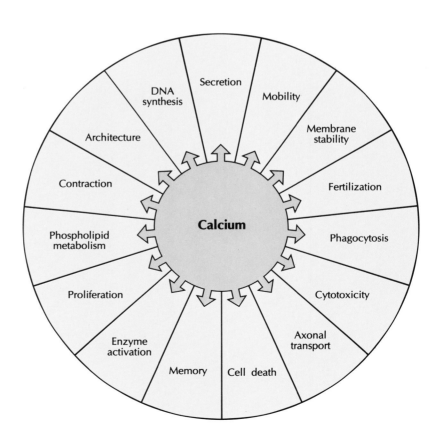

Fig. 1. Cellular events regulated by the availability and mobilization of calcium.

in its several forms, hypertension and some cardiac arrhythmias [2,3]. Definition of the sites and mechanisms of action of the calcium antagonist drugs is important both for the rational interpretation of their existing therapeutic roles and for the extension of their activities to other indications, including atherosclerosis [4,5].

Fig. 2. The calcium-dependent cycle of cell death. An initial injury (chemical or physical) produces sufficient damage to the physical or biochemical integrity of the cell to decrease energy supplies available for the ion-pumping machinery. This permits calcium entry into the cell with consequent activation of calcium-dependent phospholipases and proteases, further cell damage and eventual overload of the storage capacity and metabolic functions of the mitochondria. Cell death results.

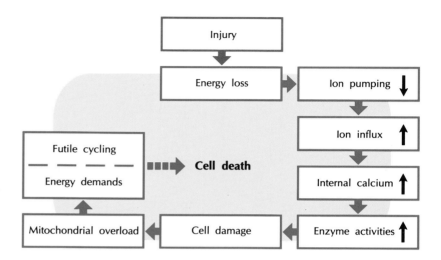

Calcium, atherosclerosis and calcium antagonists

The International Nifedipine Trial on Antiatherosclerotic Therapy (INTACT) was a multicentre, randomized, double-blind, placebo-controlled study. It demonstrated that nifedipine at a daily dose of 80 mg produced objective and significant reductions in new lesion development in the left anterior descending and left circumflex branches of the human coronary artery [6]. No regression or reduction in existing lesions was observed. A smaller trial [7] compared nifedipine, propranolol, and isosorbide dinitrate, and demonstrated that lesion progression and development were significantly reduced in the nifedipine group only. These and current trials [3,8–10] are discussed in greater detail in Chapter 3.

Experimental studies, frequently in the cholesterol-fed rabbit model of atherosclerosis [3,11–15], have focused on the role of calcium in the pathology of atherosclerosis and of calcium chelators and antagonists as therapeutic agents. Chelating agents, including ethylenediamine tetra-acetic acid (EDTA) and disodium ethane-1-hydroxy-1,1-diphosphonate (EHDP), have decreased calcium deposition and aortic cholesterol levels [15,16]. The trivalent element lanthanum is a general, but non-specific, antagonist of calcium at many sites [3] and also reduces atherogenesis in both rabbits and monkeys [16]. Such studies, while scarcely predictive of useful therapeutic regimens, have focused attention on calcium as a component of the atherosclerotic process at the level of tissue calcification and the formation of the calcified plaque.

Experimental studies during the past decade with the calcium antagonists as antiatherosclerotic agents have yielded mixed results. Henry and Bentley [17] first demonstrated that nifedipine decreased Sudan Red-stained lesions by 64% and aortic cholesterol levels by 40% in cholesterol-fed rabbits. Although the concentrations of nifedipine employed were very high, some 20 times the human therapeutic dose, the effects on blood pressure were small, suggesting that the antiatherosclerotic actions were not simply due to blood pressure reduction. Most studies with cholesterol-fed rabbits or with the Watanabe heritable hyperlipidaemic rabbit (WHHL) have used similarly high concentrations of calcium antagonists [5,11–13], but some exceptions exist where therapeutic concentrations, approximately 0.5–1.0 mg/kg, have been employed and antiatherogenic effects observed [18,19]. Not all experimental studies have shown this effect [5,13]. This is probably attributable to several factors, including the variability of lesion development in the cholesterol-fed rabbit and the time interval between induction of the atherogenic lesion or insult and the commencement of drug therapy. It may be important to start the atherogenic diet and drug treatment simultaneously [13]. This is consistent with the clinical trial data indicating that calcium antagonists may affect an early stage of the atherosclerotic process.

Calcium and cellular control

The importance of calcium for cell functions is indicated by the multiple and coordinated processes by which it is controlled, at both extra- and intracellular sites [1,3]. Such regulation (Fig. 3) is important because of the very large, approximately 10 000-fold, concentration difference between intracellular and extracellular

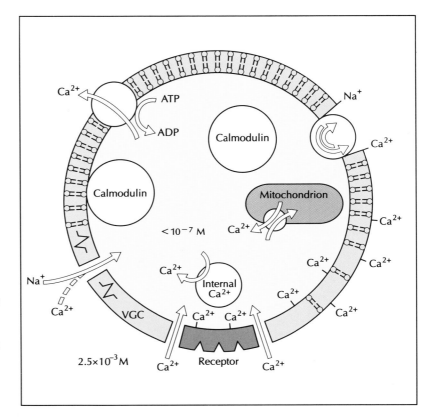

Fig. 3. Cellular calcium regulation. Intracellular calcium levels are maintained at less than 10^{-7} M in the resting state in the presence of an extracellular concentration of approximately 2.5×10^{-3} M: this represents an inwardly directed concentration gradient of some 10 000-fold. The intracellular calcium concentration rises to approximately 10^{-6} M in the excited state. Intracellular calcium levels during cell activation are controlled by a number of processes, including calcium entry through voltage-gated (VGC) and receptor-operated (ROC) channels and the sodium:calcium exchanger. Calcium may also be mobilized from the intracellular sources of mitochondria and sarcoplasmic reticulum.

concentrations. Calcium entry driven by this inwardly directed gradient represents a major cellular control point.

At the extracellular level, plasma calcium concentration is maintained by the action of a triumvirate of hormones: parathyroid, the vitamin D metabolite calcitriol, and calcitonin. Parathyroid hormone serves to mobilize bone calcium, increase kidney reabsorption and, indirectly, enhance gut absorption. Calcitriol acts similarly and is particularly important in facilitating intestinal absorption of calcium. In contrast, calcitonin facilitates deposition of calcium into bone and increases calcium excretion. These hormones respond reciprocally to changes in plasma calcium concentrations such that a decrease in calcium concentration produces an increase in parathyroid hormone and a decrease in calcitonin.

At the level of the cell, calcium movements are controlled at both plasma membrane and intracellular loci. To bring the intracellular calcium concentration up to about micromolar concentration during stimulus–response coupling, calcium is mobilized from intracellular sources, extracellular sources or both (Fig. 4). Extracellular calcium may be supplied through voltage-gated channels, receptor-operated channels and sodium : calcium exchange processes and intracellular calcium through a messenger-mediated release of calcium from the sarcoplasmic/endoplasmic reticulum (Fig. 5). These processes are biochemically and pharmacologically distinct; their relative contributions to the stimulus–response coupling event are both tissue- and stimulus-dependent.

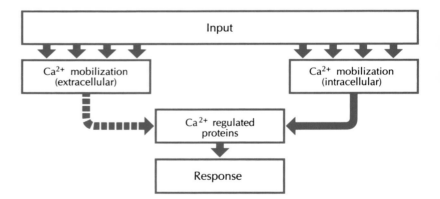

Fig. 4. The calcium requirements of cell excitation, mediated through calcium-regulated proteins, may be satisfied in response to a number of stimuli that mobilize calcium through extra- and intracellular routes.

Cellular and extracellular calcium control processes are not independent. Plasma calcium levels affect cellular excitability and membrane permeability, which both increase with decreasing calcium concentrations. Reduced plasma calcium in some essential hypertensive patients is accompanied by coordinate changes in parathyroid and calcitonin levels. These may be linked to increased intracellular calcium concentrations, increased vascular muscle tone and an enhanced sensitivity to calcium antagonists [20–22]. Vitamin D stimulates cellular calcium uptake through activation of voltage-gated calcium channels [23,24]; this could be important in vascular smooth muscle calcification [25,26].

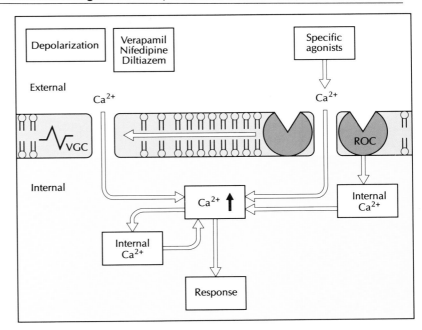

Fig. 5. Cellular calcium mobilization, depicting the several sources of mobilizable calcium and the site of action of the calcium antagonists as the voltage-gated calcium channel. In vascular smooth muscle calcium may be mobilized through the three separate pathways depicted – voltage-gated channels (VGC), receptor-operated channels (ROC) and internal stores – but only entry through the voltage-gated channel is sensitive to the calcium antagonists.

Calcium antagonists

For experimental purposes there are pharmacological agents capable of acting on calcium mobilization processes at all of the sites of calcium regulation. However, therapeutic significance attaches to one group of agents only: the calcium antagonists or calcium-channel blockers. These agents block calcium entry through one class of voltage-gated calcium channel [2,3,27,28].

The calcium antagonists are a chemically heterogeneous group of agents; they include verapamil, nifedipine and diltiazem as the original representatives of the phenylalkylamine, 1,4-dihydropyridine and benzothiazepine classes (Fig. 6). Second-generation calcium antagonists are now available, notably in the potent 1,4-dihydropyridine class, including nitrendipine, nimodipine, nisoldipine, felodipine and amlodipine (Fig. 7).

Verapamil	Nifedipine	Diltiazem

Fig. 6. Structural formulae of verapamil, nifedipine and diltiazem as the prototypical members of the phenylalkylamine, 1,4-dihydropyridine and benzothiazepine structural classes.

The discovery, elucidation of mechanism of action, classification and therapeutic use of these agents are essentially due to the pioneering work by Fleckenstein and his colleagues [2]. Their original observations established that the calcium antagonists are effective electromechanical uncouplers in the heart, that these effects mimic those of calcium removal and that inhibition is overcome by calcium-mobilizing stimuli. The application of these criteria to vascular smooth muscle served to underscore the general significance of calcium mobilization to excitation–contraction coupling in the cardiovascular system and was critical to initial considerations of the potential roles of calcium antagonists in pathological situations of calcium overload, including ischaemia and atherosclerosis [4].

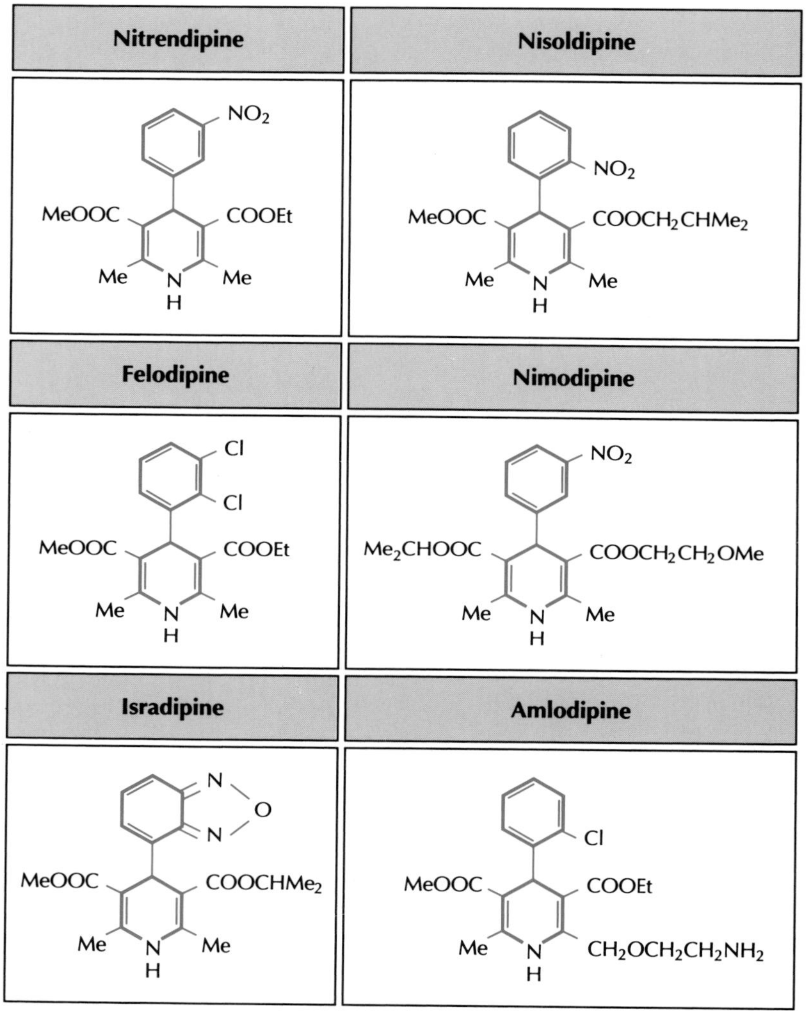

Fig. 7. Structural formulae of other members of the 1,4-dihydropyridine family of calcium antagonists.

The chemical heterogeneity of the calcium antagonists implies that they block channel function at different sites and by different mechanisms. Such conclusions are consistent with the observed quantitative and qualitative differences in therapeutic effectiveness. Biochemical observations confirm that separate binding sites exist for the several chemical classes of calcium antagonist and that these sites are linked, as depicted in the schematic representation of Fig. 8. The sites are linked both one to the other and to the permeation and gating machinery of the calcium channel by complex allosteric interactions [3,4,29,30]. These binding sites are located on a single protein, the alpha$_1$ subunit, of a heteromeric complex that expresses the major properties of channel function.

Figure 8 depicts the calcium channel as a drug-binding site or receptor. Calcium channels possess specific drug binding sites for activator and antagonist agents (and potential endogenous species). These binding sites are coupled to regulatory guanine nucleotide binding (G) proteins, and are altered in expression during disease states and chronic drug and hormone exposure. The 1,4-dihydropyridine class contains potent antagonists and activators, the latter having vasoconstrictor and positive inotropic properties. During long-term drug treatment channel numbers and function may be up- or down-regulated. Such changes have been demonstrated experimentally and clinically in cardiomyopathy, hypertension and alcoholism, and during ageing [31].

Vascular : cardiac ratio	
Verapamil	1
Diltiazem	5
Nifedipine	15

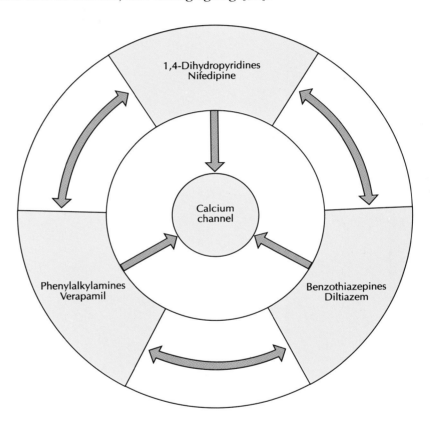

Fig. 8. The organization of calcium antagonist binding sites at the calcium channel depicted as three discrete, but linked, receptors that accommodate verapamil, nifedipine and diltiazem. This representation underscores the observation that these agents all block channel function but do so at different sites and thus exhibit different pharmacological and therapeutic properties, as indicated by the different vascular : cardiac selectivities.

The voltage-gated calcium channel family is composed of at least three major subclasses, L, T and N, which are distinguishable both electrophysiologically and pharmacologically. The **L** channels, sensitive to 1,4-dihydropyridines and other calcium antagonists, have **l**arge, **l**ong-**l**asting conductances; **T** channels give rise to **t**ransient conductances and **N** channels are confined to **n**euronal tissues. A number of distinct subtypes or isoforms of the L channel are differentially expressed in cardiac, skeletal and smooth muscle and in neurons [29,32].

The L class of channel is the major target of the existing calcium antagonists with the high-affinity interactions depicted in Figure 8. Although the available calcium antagonists are primarily cardiovascular drugs, the L channel is widely distributed in non-vascular smooth muscle, the nervous system and skeletal muscle. Because of this widespread distribution, factors that determine the selectivity of action of the calcium antagonist become very important.

In principle, selectivity derives from a number of factors, singly or in combination. The factors include pharmacokinetic properties that control tissue distribution and localization, the mode of calcium mobilization, voltage-dependent drug interactions, the pathological state of the tissue and the extent to which the calcium antagonist interacts at sites other than calcium channels. The relative vascular : cardiac activities of the calcium antagonists are one important index of selectivity, with verapamil being non-selective, diltiazem modestly selective, and nifedipine highly selective for blood vessels. These ratios not only differ between the major structural classes of antagonist, but may also differ within each class. Thus, newer 1,4-dihydropyridines may exhibit enhanced vascular : cardiac selectivity relative to nifedipine (Fig. 8). The calcium antagonists are clearly not to be regarded as a single, interchangeable set of drugs differing only quantitatively in their therapeutic activities (Fig. 9).

The clinically available calcium antagonists block potently only the L type of calcium channel. Stimuli that mobilize calcium from intracellular sources, through receptor-operated channels or through voltage-gated channels of other than the L class, are insensitive to or weakly sensitive to the calcium antagonists. Such considerations underlie the general insensitivity of skeletal muscle and neuronal systems to the antagonists: the selective sensitivity of some neuronal systems to nimodipine; the sensitivity and insensitivity, respectively, of the afferent preglomerular and the efferent postglomerular renal arterioles [33]; and the generally weak activity of the calcium antagonists as respiratory smooth muscle relaxants in asthma [34].

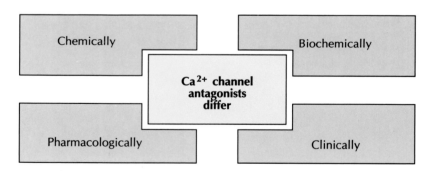

Fig. 9. Calcium antagonists differ chemically, biochemically, pharmocologically and clinically.

The interactions of the antagonists with the calcium channel are complex and subtle. The availability and affinity of binding sites depend on membrane potential and on frequency of stimulation [35]. These factors control the voltage and time-dependent distribution of resting, open and inactivated channel states (Fig. 10). Interaction with the inactivated state is facilitated by depolarization, and access to this state differs for charged and non-charged species using hydrophilic and hydrophobic pathways, respectively. This proposal accommodates the antiarrhythmic properties of verapamil (and diltiazem) and the vascular selectivity of 1,4-dihydropy-ridines [35–37].

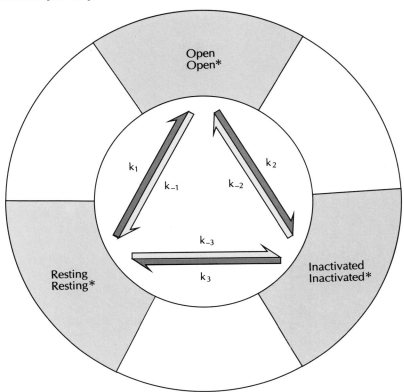

Fig. 10. The calcium channel exists in three major states – resting, open and inactivated – during which the channels are available for activation, are activated, and are in a non-activatable state, respectively. Drugs may have different affinities or access to the three states shown to generate the drug-bound states (indicated by asterisk) Calcium antagonists interact preferentially with the inactivated state and their apparent affinity is increased by depolarizing conditions. Drugs may access a binding site by 'hydrophilic' or 'hydrophobic' pathways according to the polar/non-polar balance and the charged character of the drug.

The calcium antagonists also act at a number of non-calcium channel sites. These effects appear at concentrations higher, frequently orders of magnitude higher, than those that block channel function [3,28,38]. A partial summary of these effects is presented in Fig. 11. The calcium antagonists, in particular nifedipine and the 1,4-dihydropyridines, are lipophilic agents with high partition coefficients for membranes where they may accumulate at concentrations several hundred- or thousandfold higher than the therapeutic plasma levels. Such accumulation may underscore actions at non-calcium channel sites as well as the possible effects at such sites of long-term nifedipine administration.

Modes and mechanisms of calcium antagonists in atherosclerosis

Whether the antiatherosclerotic effects of nifedipine and other calcium antagonists are through voltage-gated calcium channels or through an unrelated action is not yet known. Experimental and clinical studies with nifedipine (and the related 1,4-dihydropyridine nicardipine) suggest that it acts at an early stage of atherogenesis, rather than on established lesions.

Several processes contribute to atherogenesis, including lipid infiltration and oxidation, monocyte–macrophage accumulation, the

Ion channels		Pharmacological receptors	
Sodium Potassium Calcium (non-L type)		Acetylcholine Benzodiazepine Noradrenaline Opiates Platelet activating factor Serotonin	
Transporters		**Other**	
Sodium, potassium-ATPase Calcium-ATPase Adenosine Multiple drug resistance protein Sodium–calcium exchange		Mitochondria Platelet aggregation Renal tubules	

Fig. 11. Actions of calcium antagonists at non-calcium channel sites

release and action of chemotactic and growth factors, the formation of the 'fatty streak' and smooth muscle cell migration and proliferation (Fig. 12; reviewed in Chapter 1). Several of these processes are calcium-dependent and may be targets for calcium antagonist action. Other events may be calcium-dependent, but are not sensitive to calcium antagonists, and still other events may be both calcium-independent and calcium-antagonist-insensitive (Fig. 13). These differences find a ready explanation in the several discrete, stimulus-activated calcium mobilization pathways depicted in Fig. 5. Whether calcium mobilization occurs through the calcium-antagonist-sensitive calcium channels depends upon the cell type and the nature of the stimulus. Thus, vascular smooth muscle cells possess voltage-gated calcium channels, and contraction and migration are both calcium-dependent and calcium antagonist-sensitive. Conversely, non-excitable systems such as blood and im-

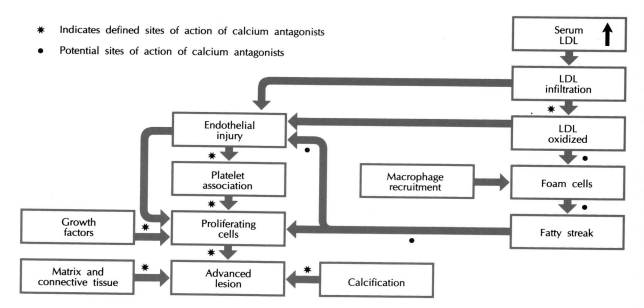

Fig. 12. Events associated with the formation of the fatty streak and with the advanced atherosclerotic lesion. The calcium antagonists may interact at one or more of these sites to exert their antiatherosclerotic actions. The possible relationships of these sites to calcium channel events are discussed in the text.

mune cells show calcium-dependent behaviour but lack voltage-gated calcium channels; calcium antagonist actions at these cells are of lower affinity at sites other than voltage-gated calcium channels, including the calcium-binding protein calmodulin and a variety of other receptors and transporters.

Atherosclerosis is accompanied by increased vascular smooth muscle reactivity to vasoconstrictor stimuli. This results from the loss of endothelium-dependent relaxation responses and the enhancement of vasoconstriction [18,39–41]. Vasodilatation by the calcium antagonists will attenuate these changes. Although the antiatherogenic actions of calcium antagonists are not simply attributable to their antihypertensive or gross haemodynamic properties, it is possible that local effects on arterial flow decrease lipid deposition at regions of low shear rates [42].

Dependent	Independent

Smooth muscle events:
    contraction
    migration
    proliferation
    transformation
	Endothelial cell function
	
	Platelet function
	
	Cholesterol processing

Neurotransmitter release	LDL processing
Growth factor release	Macrophage function

Fig. 13. Calcium-channel-dependent and independent events in atherosclerosis.

Smooth muscle cell migration from the media to the intima is an important component of early lesion development; it is both calcium-dependent and calcium-antagonist-sensitive [43,44] (Fig. 14). Smooth muscle cell migration may be part of a reinforcing cycle of vascular damage (Fig. 15); interruption by calcium antagonists will reduce endothelial cell damage, slow the recruitment of monocytes and platelets by endothelial cell factors and block the transformation of the migrated smooth muscle cells from the contractile to the synthetic phenotype. Reduction of endothelial cell damage will afford protection against increased permeability and cell death [45–47]. Smooth muscle cell proliferation in response to injury and growth factors is a calcium-dependent response sensitive to calcium antagonists. Such proliferation may be a key step in the atherogenic cascade sensitive to nifedipine [48–50]. When vascular injury was induced by balloon catheter, diltiazem, nifedipine and verapamil all reduced lesion size and reduced thymidine incorporation into DNA [48]. Platelet-derived growth factor is a potent stimulant of smooth muscle proliferation, and its mitogenic and calcium mobilizing actions are inhibited by calcium antagonists [49,51,52]. These migratory and proliferative responses of smooth muscles represent interactions of calcium antagonists at the voltage-gated channels, their primary site of action.

Several calcium-dependent processes are an integral part of the atherogenic sequence, yet are sensitive only to high concentra-

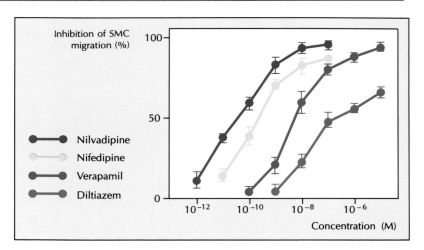

Fig. 14. Concentration–response curves for the inhibitory effects of the calcium antagonists verapamil, nifedipine, diltiazem and nilvadipine on the migration of vascular smooth muscle cells (SMC). Published by permission [44].

tions of calcium antagonists. Platelet aggregation and the release of endothelium-derived relaxing factor (EDRF) are important examples. There is, however, no evidence that endothelial cells, platelets or monocytes possess voltage-gated calcium channels, although their aggregatory, secretory and motile properties are unquestionably calcium-dependent [52,53]. Any actions of calcium antagonists on these processes must, therefore, be mediated through 'non-specific' sites, including receptors for a number of neurotransmitters and transporters (Fig. 11).

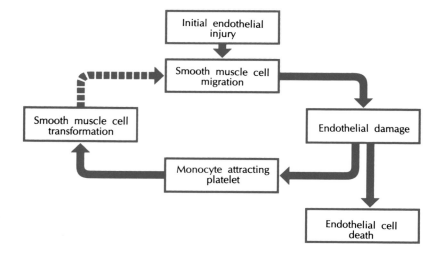

Fig. 15. A cycle in which an initial endothelial injury may permit smooth muscle cell migration to the injury site with subsequent further damage leading to endothelial cell death, the release of platelet and monocyte chemotactic factors, the phenotypic transformation of vascular smooth muscle to the proliferative state and further endothelial damage and death.

Lipid infiltration and transport are essential components of the atherogenic process. The low-density lipoprotein (LDL) receptor is a key player in the regulation of cellular cholesterol levels (Chapter 1). Calcium-calmodulin-dependent events play a role in the expression of these receptors, as calmodulin antagonists stimulate receptor synthesis in human skin fibroblasts and aortic muscle cells. High concentrations of diltiazem and verapamil, but not nifedipine, are effective [54–56]. This is consistent with a calmodulin interaction that demands an amphiphilic molecule. Isradipine, a 1,4-dihydropyridine related to nifedipine, at therapeutically effective concentrations inhibited LDL entry into vascular smooth muscle of the cholesterol-fed rabbit [57]. The effects, although not large, were greatest when the endothelial lining was damaged and were accompanied by an increased prostacyclin production. As verapamil and diltiazem are also reported to enhance the anti-atherosclerotic activity of a prostacyclin analogue [58], an action of calcium antagonists on the synthesis or action of prostacyclin is possible.

The atheromatous fatty streak is characterized by foam cells. These cells are macrophages recruited into the intima which take up oxidized or chemically modified LDL through the type I and type II scavenger receptors [59,60]. Oxidized LDL is believed to be a major contributor to the development of the atherosclerotic lesion. There is no evidence that calcium antagonists interact directly with either the LDL receptor or the scavenger receptors, but calcium antagonists may block formation of oxidized LDL through antioxidant actions. The three major antagonist classes inhibit superoxide production in neutrophils, prevent phospholipid oxidation and protect against hydrogen peroxide-induced increases in endothelial cell permeability [48,61,62]. The antioxidant effects of the calcium antagonists are at high concentrations and are not at calcium channels. However, these effects could be important to the antiatherosclerotic actions of calcium antagonists, interrupting foam cell formation and preventing other effects of oxidized LDL that contribute to the atherogenic process, including inactivation of EDRF, cytotoxicity on endothelial cells, chemoattraction of monocytes and macrophage motility [57,63,64].

Calcium antagonists may modify cholesterol ester metabolism. Nifedipine and verapamil, but not diltiazem, inhibit cholesterol ester deposition in macrophages [65] and nifedipine promotes cholesterol efflux from cholesterol-laden macrophages by a HDL-independent mechanism [66]. Additionally, nifedipine increases cholesteryl ester hydrolase activity in lipid-loaded cultured vascular smooth muscle cells and decreases cholesterol content [67]. An increase in cholesteryl ester hydrolase activity occurs in human arterial smooth muscle cells from people chronically treated with nifedipine and diltiazem and a reduction in both free and esterified cholesterol content occurs. This effect occurs at therapeutic concentrations and may be a significant contributor to the antiatherosclerotic profile of nifedipine [68]. The relationship of this process to calcium channel activity remains to be established.

Future prospects

The antiatherosclerotic activities of nifedipine and other calcium antagonists in experimental and clinical situations are of scientific and therapeutic significance. What remains to be determined is whether the same mechanisms are responsible for the experimental and the clinical effects. Although we understand how calcium antagonists act on voltage-gated calcium channels to produce their cardiovascular effects, it is not clear whether this action also accounts for the antiatherosclerotic mechanism. Both experimental and clinical studies suggest that calcium antagonists act at an early stage of atherosclerosis. It is important to distinguish actions at channels from actions at other sites and current experimental studies are devised to make this distinction. This should permit the design of agents with enhanced antiatherosclerotic activity and the confirmation of a new therapeutic direction for the calcium antagonists.

References

1. Campbell AK:*Intracellular Calcium. Its Universal Role as Regulator.* New York and London: Wiley, 1983.
2. Fleckenstein A: *Calcium Antagonism in Heart and Smooth Muscle. Experimental Facts and Therapeutic Prospects.* New York and London: Wiley, 1983.
3. Janis RA, Silver PJ, Triggle DJ: Drug action and cellular calcium regulation. *Adv Drug Res* 1987; 16:309–591.
4. Triggle DJ: Calcium antagonists. History and perspective. *Stroke* 1990; 21(suppl IV):49–58.
5. Triggle DJ: Calcium antagonists and atherosclerosis. *Drugs Today* 1991 (in press).
6. Lichtlen PR, Hugenholtz, PG, Rafflenbeul W, Hecker W, Jost S, Nikutter P, Deckers JW: Retardation of coronary artery disease by the calcium channel blocker nifedipine: results of the INTACT study (International Nifedipine Trial on Antiatherosclerotic Therapy). *Cardiovasc Drugs* 1990; 4: 1047–1068.
7. Loaldi A, Polese A, Montorsi P, DeCesare N, Fabbiocchi F, Ravagnani P, Guazzi MD: Comparison of nifedipine, propranolol and isosorbide dinitrate on angiographic progression and regression of coronary arterial narrowings in angina pectoris. *Am J Cardiol* 1989; 64:433–439.
8. Waters D, Lesperance J, Fracetich M, Causey D, Theroux P, Chiang Y-K, Hudon G, Lemarbre L, Reitman M, Joyal M, Gosselin G, Dryda I, Macer J, Havel RJ: A controlled clinical trial to assess the effect of a calcium channel blocker on the progression of coronary atherosclerosis. *Circulation* 1990: 82:1940–1953.
9. Grimm RH, Flack JM, Byington R, Bond G, Brugger S: A comparison of antihypertensive drug effects on the progression of extracranial carotid atherosclerosis. The Multicenter Isradipine Diuretic Atherosclerotic Study (MIDAS). *Drugs* 1990; 40 (suppl 2):38–43.
10. Schneider WJ, Kober G, Roebruck P, Noack H, Alle M, Ciestinstii G, Reifart N, Kaltenbach M: Retardation of development and progression of coronary atherosclerosis: a new indication for calcium antagonists. *Eur J Clin Pharmacol* 1990; 39 (suppl 1):17–23.
11. Henry PD: Antiatherogenic effects of calcium channel blockers: possible mechanisms of action. *Cardiovasc Drugs Ther* 1990; 4 (suppl 5):1015–1020.
12. Weinstein DB, Heider JG: Antiatherogenic properties of calcium antagonists. *Am J Med 1989;* 86 (suppl 4A):27–32.
13. Jackson CL, Bush RC, Bowyer DE: Mechanism of antiatherogenic action of calcium antagonists. *Atherosclerosis* 1989; 80:17–26.
14. Henry PD: Antiatherogenic effects of calcium-channel blockers: possible mechanisms of action. *Cardiovasc Drugs Ther* 1990; 4:1015–1020.
15. Kjeldsen K, Stender S: Calcium antagonists and experimental atherosclerosis. *Proc Soc Exp Biol Med* 1991; 191:219–228.
16. Kramsch DM: Calcium antagonists and atherosclerosis. *Adv Exp Med Biol* 1985; 183:323–348.
17. Henry PD, Bentley KI: Suppression of atherogenesis in cholesterol-fed rabbits treated with nifedipine. *J Clin Invest* 1981; 68:1366–1369.
18. Habib JB, Bossailer C, Wells S, Williams C, Morrisett JD, Henry PD: Preservation of endothelium-dependent vascular relaxation in cholesterol-fed rabbit by treatment with the calcium blocker PN 200 110. *Circ Res* 1986; 58: 305–309.
19. Nayler WG, Dillon JS, Panagiotopoulos S, Sturrock, WJ: Dihydropyridines and the ischemic myocardium. In *Proceedings of the 6th International Adalat Symposium: New Therapy of Ischemic Heart Disease and Hypertension* edited by Lichtlen PR. Amsterdam: Elsevier, 1986; 386–397.
20. Young EW, Bukoski RD, McCarron D: Calcium metabolism in experimental hypertension. *Proc Soc Exp Med Biol* 1988; 187:123–141.
21. Resnick LM, Laragh JH: Renin, calcium metabolism and the pathophysiologic basis of antihypertensive therapy. *Am J Cardiol* 1985; 56:68H–74H.
22. Resnick LM: Uniformity and diversity of calcium metabolism in hypertension. A conceptual framework. *Am J Med* 1987; 82 (suppl 1B):16–26.
23. Inoue T, Kawashima H: 1,25-Dihydroxyvitamin D3 stimulates $45Ca^{2+}$-uptake by cultured vascular smooth muscle cells derived from rat aorta. *Biochem Biophys Res Commun* 1988; 152: 1388–1394.
24. Tornquist K, Tashjian AH: Dual actions of 1,25-dihydroxycholecalciferol on intracellular Ca^{2+} in GH_4C_1 cells: evidence for effects on voltage-operated Ca^{2+} channels and Na^+/Ca^{2+} exchange. *Endocrinology* 1989; 124:2765–2776.
25. Fleckenstein A, Frey M, Zorn G, Fleckenstein-Grün G: The role of calcium in the pathogenesis of experimental atherosclerosis. *Trends Pharmacol Sci* 1987; 8:496–501.
26. Fleckenstein A, Frey M, Thimm F, Fleckenstein-Grün G: Excessive mural calcium overload – a predominant causal factor in the development of stenosing coronary plaques in humans. *Cardiovasc Drugs Ther* 1990; 4:1005–1014.
27. Triggle DJ: Calcium Antagonists. In *Cardiovascular Pharmacology* edited by Antonnaccio. New York: Raven Press: 107–160, 1990.
28. Godfraind T, Miller R, Wibo M: Calcium antagonism and calcium entry blockade. *Pharmacol Rev* 1986; 38: 321–416.
29. Catterall WA: Structure and function of voltage-sensitive ion channels. *Science* 1988; 242:50–61.
30. McKenna E, Koch WJ, Slish DF, Schwartz A: Towards an understanding of the dihydropyridine-sensitive calcium channel. *Biochem Pharmacol* 1990; 39: 1145–1150.
31. Ferrante J, Triggle DJ: Drug- and disease-induced regulation of the voltage-dependent calcium channel. *Pharmacol Rev* 1990; 42:29–44.
32. Bean BP: Classes of calcium channels in vertebrate cells. *Physiol Rev* 1989; 51: 367–384.
33. Loutzenhiser R, Epstein M: The renal hemodynamic effects of calcium antagonists. In *Calcium Antagonists and the Kidney* edited by Epstein M, Loutzenhiser R. Philadelphia: Hanley and Belfus, 1990.
34. Ahmed T: Calcium channel blockers. *Immunol Allergy Clinics North Am* 1990; 10.3:515–530.
35. Hondeghem LM, Katzung BG: Antiarrhythmic agents: the modulated receptor mechanism of action of sodium and calcium channel blocking drugs. *Annu Rev Pharmacol Toxicol* 1985; 24:387–423.
36. Godfraind T, Morel N, Wibo M: Modulation of the action of calcium antagonists in arteries. *Blood Vessels* 1990; 27:184–196.
37. Nelson MT, Potlack JB, Worley JF, Standen NB: Calcium channels, potassium channels and voltage-dependence of arterial smooth muscle tone. *Am J Physiol* 1990; 259:C3–C18.
38. Janis RA, Triggle DJ: Drugs acting on calcium channels. In *Calcium Channels*

edited by Hurwitz L. Boca Raton: CRC Press (in press).

39. Cohen RA, Zitnay KM, Haudenschild CC, Cunningham LD: Loss of selective endothelial cell vasoactive functions caused by hypercholesterolemia in pig coronary arteries. *Circ Res* 1988; 63:903–910.

40. Merkel LA, Rivera LM, Bilder GE, Perrone MH: Differential alteration of vascular reactivity in rabbit aorta with modest elevation of serum cholesterol. *Circ Res* 1990; 67:550–555.

41. Tagawa H, Tomoike H, Nakamura M: Putative mechanism of the impairment of endothelium-dependent relaxation of the aorta with atheromatous plaque in heritable hyperlipidemic rabbits. *Circ Res* 1991; 68:330–337.

42. Woolf N: Atherosclerosis and its genesis. In *Atheroma*. London: Science Press, 1990:1.1–1.68

43. Nakao J, Ito H, Ooyama T, Chang W-C, Murota S-I: Calcium dependency of aortic smooth muscle cell migration induced by 12-L-hydroxy-5,8,10,14-eicosatetraenoic acid. *Atherosclerosis* 1983; 46:309–319.

44. Nomoto A, Hirosumi J, Sekiguchi C, Mutoh S, Yamaguchi I, Aoki H: Anti-atherogenic activity of FR 34235 (nilvadipine), a new potent calcium antagonist. *Atherosclerosis* 1987; 64: 255–261.

45. Strohschneider T, Betz E: Densitometric measurement of increased endothelial permeability in arteriosclerotic plaques and inhibition of permeability under the influence of two antagonists. *Atherosclerosis* 1989; 75:135–144.

46. Yamada Y, Yokota M, Furumichi T, Furui H, Yamauchi K, Saito H: Protective effects of calcium channel blockers on hydrogen peroxide induced increases in endothelial permeability. *Cardiovasc Res* 1990; 24:993–997.

47. Lefer AM, Sedar AW: Endothelial alterations in hypercholesterolemia and atherosclerosis. *Pharmacol Rev* 1991;23:1–12.

48. Jackson CL, Bush RC, Bowyer DE: Inhibitory effects of calcium antagonists on balloon catheter-induced arterial smooth muscle cell proliferation and lesion size. *Atherosclerosis* 1988; 69:115–122.

49. Block LH, Emmons RR, Vogt E, Sachinidis A, Vetter W, Hoppe J: Ca^{2+} channel blockers inhibit the action of recombinant platelet-derived growth in vascular smooth muscle cells. *Proc Natl Acad Sci USA* 1989; 86:2388–2392.

50. Nilsson J, Sjolund M, Palmberg L, von Euler AM, Jonzon B, Thyberg J: The calcium antagonist nifedipine inhibits arterial smooth muscle cell proliferation. *Atherosclerosis* 1985; 58:109–122.

51. Libby P, Warner SJC, Salomon RN, Birinyi LK: Production of platelet-derived growth factor-like mitogens by smooth muscle cells from human atheroma. *N Engl J Med* 1988; 318:1493–1498.

52. Pannocchia A, Praloran N, Ardvino C, Dora ND, Bazzan M, Schinco P, Buraglio M, Pileri A, Tamponi G: Absence of (−) (3H)desmethoxyverapamil binding sites on human platelets and lack of evidence for voltage-dependent calcium channels. *Eur J Pharmacol* 1987; 142:83–91.

53. Takeda K, Klepper M: Voltage-dependent and agonist-activated ionic currents in vascular endothelial cells: a review. *Blood Vessels* 1990; 27:169–183.

54. Filipovic I, Buddecke E: Calmodulin antagonists stimulate LDL receptor synthesis in human skin fibroblasts. *Biochim Biophys Acta* 1986; 876:124–132.

55. Corsini A, Granata A, Fumagalli R, Paoletti R: Calcium antagonists and low density lipoprotein metabolism by human fibroblasts and by human hepatoma cell line HEPG2. *Pharmacol Res Commun* 1986; 16:1–16.

56. Paoletti R, Bernini F: A new generation of calcium antagonists and their role in atherosclerosis. *Am J Cardiol* 1990; 66:28–31.

57. Sizinger H, Lupattelli G, Virgolini I, Gerakakis A, Fitscha P, Molinari E, Angelberger P: Isradipine, a calcium entry blocker, decreases vascular (^{125}I)low-density lipoprotein entry in hypercholesterolemic rabbits. *J Cardiovasc Pharmacol* 1991; 17:546–550.

58. Akopov SE, Orekhov AN, Tertov VV, Khashimov KA, Gabrielyan ES, Smirnov VN: Stable analogs of prostacyclin and thromboxane A2 display contradictory influences on atherosclerotic properties of cells cultured from human aorta. *Atherosclerosis* 1988; 72:245–248.

59. Steinberg D, Parthasrathy S, Carew TE, Khoo JC, Witztum JL: Beyond cholesterol: modifications of low-density lipoprotein that increase its atherogenicity. *N Engl J Med* 1989; 320:915–924.

60. Kodama T, Freeman M, Rohrer L, Zabrecky M, Matsudaira P, Krieger M: Type I macrophage scavenger receptor contains alpha-helical and collagen-like coiled coils. *Nature* 1990; 343:531–535.

61. Irita K, Fujita I, Takeshige K, Minakami S, Yoshitake J: Calcium channel antagonist induced inhibitory superoxide production in human neutrophils. Mechanisms independent of antagonizing calcium influx. *Biochem Pharmacol* 1986; 35: 3465–3471.

62. Shridi F, Robak J: The influence of calcium channel blockers on superoxide anions. *Pharmacol Res Commun* 1988; 20:13–21.

63. Quinn MT, Parthasarathy S, Fong LG, Steinberg D: Oxidatively modified low density lipoprotein: a potential role in recruitment and retention of monocytes/macrophages during atherogenesis. *Proc Natl Acad Sci USA* 1987; 84:2995–2998.

64. Quinn MT, Parthasarathy S, Steinberg D: Endothelial cell-defined chemotactic activity for mouse peritoneal macrophages and the effects of modified low density lipoproteins. *Proc Natl Acad Sci USA* 1985; 82:5949–5953.

65. Daugherty A, Rateri DL, Schonfeld G, Sobel BE: Inhibition of cholesteryl ester hydrolysis in macrophages by calcium entry blockers. *Br J Pharmacol* 1987; 91:113–118.

66. Schmitz G, Robernek H, Beuck M, Krause R, Schurek A, Niemann R: Ca^{2+} antagonists and ACAT inhibitors promote cholesterol efflux from macrophages by different mechanisms. I. Characterization of cellular lipid metabolism. *Arteriosclerosis* 1988; 8:46–56.

67. Etingin OR, Hajjer DP: Nifedipine increases cholesteryl ester hydrolytic activity in lipid-laden rabbit arterial smooth muscle cells. A possible mechanism for its antiatherogenic effects. *J Clin Invest* 1985; 75:1554–1558.

68. Etingin OR, Hajjer DP: Calcium channel blockers enhance cholesteryl ester hydrolysis and decrease total cholesterol accumulation in human aortic tissue. *Circ Res* 1990; 66:185–190.

3 Current clinical evaluation of the role of the calcium channel antagonists in atherosclerosis

Introduction

Atherosclerosis is the major cause of chronic disease and death in western countries, accounting for almost 50% of deaths in those below 65 years of age [1]. The term atherosclerosis is derived from the Greek 'athere' and 'scler', meaning porridge and hard, respectively. These words, 'hard porridge', are a reasonable description of the atheromatous plaques that develop in the walls of the arteries of humans. Atherosclerosis is manifest as many clinical entities but most commonly affects the arteries in the brain, causing stroke, or in the heart, where atherosclerosis develops in the coronary arteries. The presence of atherosclerosis in the arteries of the heart leads to the entity called coronary artery disease. The major clinical consequences are myocardial infarction, angina pectoris, sudden death, and heart failure (Fig. 1)

- Myocardial infarction
- Stable angina
- Unstable angina
- Increased vascular constriction
- Episodic chest pain without infarction
- Sudden death
- Heart failure

Fig. 1. Syndromes associated with atheroma in coronary arteries.

Major advances in the prevention, early detection, and treatment of coronary artery disease have been made in the last few years. The use of thrombolytic drugs has resulted in a reduction in the 1 year mortality from myocardial infarction [2,3]. The use of coronary artery bypass surgery and percutaneous angioplasty, and the availability of drugs such as the nitrates in new formulations, beta blockers and the calcium antagonists have done much to alleviate the symptoms of patients with angina pectoris. New methods are emerging for the early detection of atheroma. Nuclear magnetic resonance techniques and fast computerized tomography may provide the means not just to measure coronary blood flow in the presence of known atheromatous disease in the coronary arteries, but the ability to detect small lesions and to provide information on the nature of these lesions, thus enabling the physician to predict the likely importance of particular lesions.

To convert cholesterol values from mmol/l to mg/dl, multiply by 38.7

Despite these advances, the prevention of the sequelae of coronary artery disease has remained problematic and often controversial [4–9]. Public health measures are widely advocated for prevention

[10,11]. Interventional or medical treatments are used to treat the manifestations of the disease. A different approach would be to introduce measures which delayed, prevented, or even reversed the enlargement or breakdown of the atheromatous plaques in the coronary arteries. This has been attempted with drug therapies or by alterations of the diet aimed at reducing the blood cholesterol [12]. Recently, a similar approach has been undertaken using the calcium antagonist drugs [13,14].

The calcium antagonists were discovered in the 1960s and introduced into clinical medicine in the 1970s. During the 1980s they gained wide acceptance for the treatment of angina pectoris and hypertension (Fig. 2). Their use in other conditions such as arrhythmias, stroke, claudication, and hypertrophic cardiomyopathy is more controversial. In unstable angina, acute myocardial infarction and heart failure, calcium antagonists have not in general been shown to be advantageous [15–18] although certain subsets of patients may derive considerable benefit [19–21]. During the 1980s a considerable amount of evidence emerged from animal experimentation to suggest that these drugs might influence the growth of atheromatous plaques [22,23]. This resulted in two large studies where an attempt was made to determine whether the use of calcium antagonists delayed progression or even caused regression of atheromatous lesions in the coronary arteries of human beings [13,14].

Fig. 2. Cardiovascular applications of calcium antagonists.

Established indications	Uncertain indications
1. Angina pectoris	1. Unstable angina
2. Unstable angina	2. Acute myocardial infarction
3. Arrhythmias	3. Heart failure
4. Hypertension	4. Stroke
5. Hypertrophic cardiomyopathy	5. Intermittent claudication

The nature of atheroma in man

Although much useful work on atheroma has been undertaken in animal models, the disease in animals differs in many respects from that in humans. Animal models often have cholesterol blood concentrations higher than those occurring in humans. The histopathology of the lesions is not always characteristic of the lesions in humans. The natural history of the abnormalities in animals is more rapid than in humans. Perhaps the major lesson to be learnt from animal models is that the potential for the reversal of atheromatous disease does exist [22,23]. Regression of atheromatous lesions by diet or drugs has been shown in many animal species.

In humans the abnormality has several features that can never be mimicked by animal models, such as slow onset (over 30 years), manifestation around 50 years of age, the complex histology of the plaque, and the relation to metabolic abnormalities including lipids, the coagulation cascade, carbohydrate metabolism and sex hormones. There is evidence that atheroma is related to neonatal and postnatal nutrition [24].

Regression of atheroma by the use of calcium antagonists has been demonstrated in animal models, although the mechanism is unclear [22,23]. The calcium antagonists were originally described as a group of drugs which inhibited the calcium channel in the surface membrane (sarcolemma) of heart muscle and vascular smooth muscle. They were thought to have a rather specific action. However, they may influence platelet function, prevent endothelial cell damage, inhibit cell proliferation, suppress tissue mineralization, interfere with cell migration and the laying down of the extracellular matrix, and the accumulation of intracellular lipids (Fig. 3). A drug with so many actions would be expected to have a number of side effects in humans. The calcium antagonists are, however, remarkably free of side effects. Ankle oedema and flushing occur rarely.

Fig. 3. Mechanisms for the advantageous effects of calcium antagonists on atheromatous plaques in man.

> 1. Lowering of blood pressure
> 2. Altered stress in arterial wall
> 3. Reduced blood lipids
> 4. Interference with platelet activity
> 5. Prevention of damage of endothelium
> 6. Inhibition of smooth muscle cell proliferation
> 7. Prevention of calcium deposition in plaques
> 8. Effect on extracellular structure of matrix in plaque
> 9. Inhibition of growth factors
> 10. Prevention of free radical activity
> 11. Delay in cell necrosis by prevention of calcium overload

The origins and natural history of atherosclerosis in animals and man (Fig. 4) are discussed in the preceding chapters. Many factors interact and it is not possible yet to describe accurately the progression from early lesions to the established atheromatous plaque. Injury of the cell membrane, lipid infiltration, encrustation with platelets, and malfunction of many cell types may all be involved. Atheroma is believed to begin as a fatty streak in the cell membrane. Some of these streaks may spontaneously resolve whereas others proceed to the formation of atheromatous lesions over a period of many years.

Fig. 4. Theories for the aetiology of atheroma.

> - Response to injury (Virchow, 1856)
> - Infiltration with lipids (Anitschkow and Chalatow, 1913)
> - Platelet adherence and layering (Duguid, 1949)
> - Malfunction or activation of other cell types
>   Endothelial cells
>   Platelets
>   Monocytes/macrophages
>   Lymphocytes

Not only is the enlargement of an atheromatous plaque a complex process but the mechanisms by which lesions lead to clinical syndromes are many. If an atheromatous plaque remains with a smooth surface then the likely clinical problem will be stable angina pectoris which may progress only slowly over many years. Obstruction of the lumen of the artery by a fixed obstruction is not the most dangerous manifestation of coronary artery atherosclerosis. Sudden death and myocardial infarction are usually associated with an unstable plaque [25–27] that ruptures, allowing blood elements to be exposed to the raw surface of the interior of the plaque and notably to collagen. Platelets accumulate at this site and a thrombosis develops. Myocardial infarction can result [27]. The rupture of plaques is probably a common event and not all ruptured plaques inevitably result in thrombosis of sufficient magnitude to occlude the coronary artery and bring about myocardial infarction. Indeed, the rupturing of a plaque and the accumulation of platelets on the surface of the plaque may be an important mechanism for the growth of plaques, which often show evidence of layering and rapid growth interspersed with periods of quiescence. Abnormalities of the clotting system may be critical for the manifestation of a ruptured plaque as a clinical event. In that case the plaque rupture would be the substrate for myocardial infarction but a propensity to thrombosis the critical abnormality. The plaques which rupture tend to be those which are lipid-rich rather than fibrotic and calcified. The site of the rupture is often where the fibrous cap is not firmly attached to the smooth muscle wall because of the presence of lipid [27]. These ideas lead to the possibility that techniques such as magnetic resonance imaging may be able to identify those plaques which are most likely to rupture and the lipid-laden plaques which are most likely to regress with treatment.

Lipids, cholesterol, risk factors and atheroma

The occurrence of atheroma in coronary arteries and clinical events arising from the presence of atheroma have been associated with many risk factors. Of these the most important are sex, family history, smoking, hypertension, abnormalities of lipids, abnormal carbohydrate metabolism, and obesity. Sex and family history are not true risk factors since they are unalterable. Recently emphasis has been placed on cholesterol, high and-low-density lipoproteins and newly discovered lipoproteins such as lipoprotein(a). The importance of the clotting system and in particular fibrinogen and factor VII has been emphasized [28]. The prevention of coronary artery disease by the reversal of the other factors has been the subject of numerous studies and a vast effort on the part of physicians, epidemiologists, and health workers. The results have often given rise to controversy, and doctors have been the worst advocates of their findings. The tendency to concentrate on one single aspect of the disease has sometimes led to exaggerated claims which have eagerly been seized on by critics. Thus, in September 1989, Thomas J. Moore in the *Atlantic Monthly* [29] wrote an article entitled 'The cholesterol myth – Lowering your cholesterol is next to impossible with diet, and often dangerous with drugs – and it won't make you live any longer'. Nigel Hawkes in *The Times* (London) [30] of 22 September 1990 writes under the title 'Leave us to our chips: this hectoring is even worse'. Such articles undoubtedly reflect the opinion of a substantial section of the public who read about conflicting information and opinions and who also may not wish to alter their style of life, thus welcoming any evidence of confusion amongst doctors on this issue. The data as presented to the public do confuse, often as a result of injudicious statements or exaggerated claims by the medical profession. The medical profession and other health workers need to have a clearer message. The key advice, on which there is almost no disagreement, is shown in Fig. 5. Other aspects of the prevention of coronary events are still being debated. For example, how or whether to screen the population is uncertain [31,32]. The appropriate mechanism for assessing how to distribute limited health resources between acute health care for heart disease and prevention of heart disease is not established. The value of drug therapy for lipid disorders, other than the severe lipid disorders, is still under investigation.

- Stop smoking.
- Detect and treat hypertension.
- Avoid obesity.
- Vary the diet. Moderate fat intake from animal sources.
- Exercise regularly.

Fig. 5. General advice for the prevention of ischaemic heart disease.

A large amount of data has accumulated in the last decade on the role of lipid metabolism and its relation to the occurrence of acute coronary disorders. Blood cholesterol levels are related to the increased likelihood of a coronary event or death (Fig. 6). The Framingham study [33] has shown over 30 years that the blood cholesterol concentration in those under 50 years correlates with overall and cardiovascular mortality. An odd feature of the study was that if the cholesterol fell in the first 14 years of observation mortality was increased. Many large studies have been reported where an attempt has been made to alter the mortality from or occurrence of coronary events by altering risk factors, changing diet, or drug treatment. These have been reviewed in several meta-analyses, which do not always come to the same conclusions [12,34,35]. It is agreed that the occurrence of coronary events is reduced by both drugs and diet in both primary and secondary trials [12,34,35]. Furthermore, the effect is greater if the initial cholesterol concentration is high. Total mortality in an analysis of trials involving up to 103 598 patients may be altered in some subgroups of patients but not in others [12]. Indeed, in patients with a low total cholesterol level there is a possibility that mortality is increased and that lowering cholesterol can increase deaths either from cancer or because of an altered behaviour pattern [36,37].

Those who wish to denigrate the role of lipids in heart disease will point to the failure to show a reduction in overall mortality, the increased mortality at low blood cholesterol concentrations, the lack of data in women, the small effect on longevity, the side effects associated with diet or drug therapy, the expense, and the small effect on coronary events.

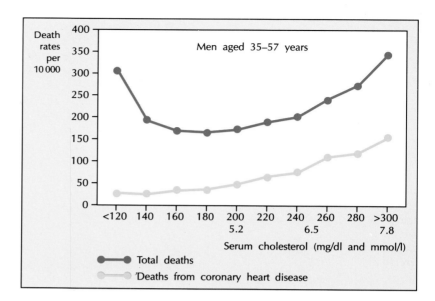

Fig. 6. Age-adjusted death rates over 6 years per 10 000 people. Adapted by permission (Iso H *et al. N Engl J Med* 1989; **320**:904–910).

Those who favour the cholesterol hypothesis will point to the inadequate size of trials to detect an effect on mortality, the desirable reduction on coronary events, the fact that these trials showed an effect although they were short (5 years approximately) and began in middle-aged people, many of whom would already have had established but undetected coronary heart disease. A most persuasive argument is the correlation between the decline in the occurrence of coronary heart disease and the size of the reduction in blood cholesterol concentration (Figs 7 and 8).

The health problems relating to coronary heart disease have not been solved by these trials. A more useful way forward may be the identification of specific subgroups of patients at risk by the detection of genetic characteristics or lipid profiles. This may allow the identification of smaller groups of patients with known risk that can then be modified by an intervention.

The second approach is to use the coronary anatomy as a surrogate of the existence of coronary heart disease. For the reasons given above, the existence of atheromatous lesions in the coronary arteries may only be a substrate, not a cause, of a coronary event. Nevertheless, the detection of lesions in the coronary arteries and the demonstration that the site of the lesions could be reversed would be persuasive information favouring the further evaluation of an intervention. The advantage of such an approach is that trials can be undertaken on relatively small numbers of patients.

The efficacy of an intervention directed towards the reduction of coronary events could be tested by investigating the effect of the intervention either on the occurrence of those events (Fig. 9) or on a surrogate, namely the presence of the atheromatous plaque in the coronary artery.

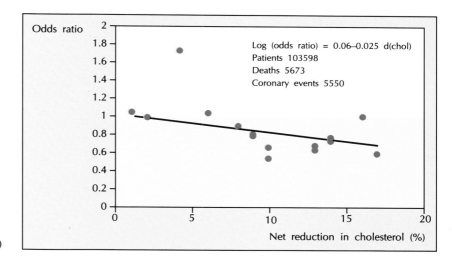

Fig. 7. Coronary heart disease incidence and reduction of cholesterol in 16 trials. Adapted by permission (Holme *Circulation* 1990; **82**:1916–1924.)

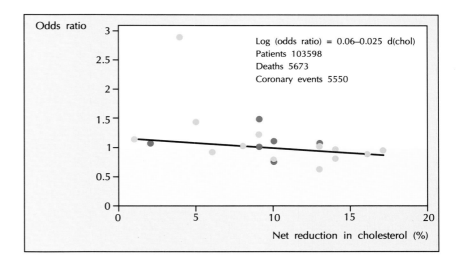

Fig. 8. Total mortality and reduction of cholesterol in 19 trials. Adapted by permission (Holme *Circulation* 1990; **82**:1916–1924.)

Current clinical use of calcium antagonists

The role of calcium antagonists in the prevention of atheroma can be assessed either by direct measurement of the size of the atheromatous plaque or by the effect on the clinical endpoints of coronary artery disease. In general, calcium antagonists are now established as treatment for angina pectoris and hypertension (Fig. 2). The use of these drugs in other clinical conditions is more controversial. The calcium antagonists have been shown to be remarkably free of side effects, the major ones being reversible ankle oedema and dizziness or headaches. This latter symptom may be related to the pharmacokinetics of the drug. Most calcium antagonists have a very short half-life. The onset of action may be rapid. Newer calcium antagonists or new formulations of older calcium antagonists

> **Total mortality**
>   Diet and drugs have similar effects
>   Secondary prevention is more effective than primary
>   Advantage is gained only if cholesterol reduced by more than 8%
>   Single and multiple factor trials are no different
>
> **Incidence of coronary heart disease**
>   Primary and secondary trials do not differ
>   Drugs are marginally more effective than diet
>   Greater benefit is gained if initial cholesterol is high
>
> 10 3598 patients, 5673 deaths, 5550 coronary events

Fig. 9. Effects of cholesterol reduction from 19 trials. Adapted by permission (Holme *Circulation* 1990; **82**:1916–1924).

have a longer duration of action and a slower onset of effect. This is an important point. The action of the calcium antagonists does seem to be related to the presence of the drug in the blood. If there are large peaks in concentrations and troughs between dosage the clinical effect of the drug will appear to be variable.

Haemodynamic properties of calcium antagonists

The mechanism of action of the calcium antagonists in effort-related angina pectoris is linked to their effects on the haemodynamics of the heart (Fig. 10). In vasospastic angina the drugs act directly on the smooth muscle of the coronary arteries. The effects on the vasculature increase blood flow to the myocardium and a minor negative inotropic effect reduces oxygen consumption by the myocardium. The systemic effects on the arteries and veins increase the perfusion pressure marginally, assuming the fall in end-diastolic pressure is greater than the fall of diastolic arterial pressure. There are two potentially harmful effects of the calcium antagonists: an excessive fall of blood pressure and reflex tachycardia.

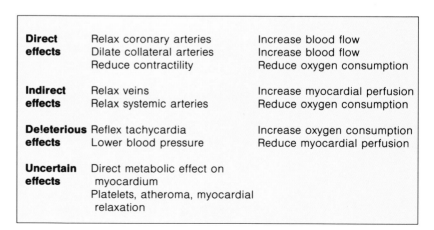

Direct effects	Relax coronary arteries	Increase blood flow
	Dilate collateral arteries	Increase blood flow
	Reduce contractility	Reduce oxygen consumption
Indirect effects	Relax veins	Increase myocardial perfusion
	Relax systemic arteries	Reduce oxygen consumption
Deleterious effects	Reflex tachycardia	Increase oxygen consumption
	Lower blood pressure	Reduce myocardial perfusion
Uncertain effects	Direct metabolic effect on myocardium	
	Platelets, atheroma, myocardial relaxation	

Fig. 10. Haemodynamic and cellular effects of calcium antagonists.

Calcium antagonists in ischaemic heart disease

Animal experiments had indicated that the calcium antagonists would be of major benefit in the treatment of myocardial infarction and unstable angina [38]. The reasons for an expected protection of the ischaemic myocardium are shown in Fig. 11. Clinical experience has been disappointing (Figs 12–15). Two more recent trials have, however, been more encouraging [19–21]. In the Multicentre Diltiazem Postinfarction Trial (MDPIT) study [19,20] patients received 240 mg/day of diltiazem. After a mean observation period of 25 months the mortality rate and incidence of coronary events were unchanged. However, there was a marked difference if patients with heart failure were excluded. In the remaining subgroup a reduction of mortality was evident. As many as 55% of patients were receiving a beta blocker and the combination of a beta blocker and diltiazem may not have been advantageous. The second trial to be reported [21] recently was the Danish Verapamil Infarction Trial II (DAVIT II). In this study 1775 patients were randomized to placebo or verapamil 360 mg/day. Treatment began in the second week after a myocardial infarct and continued for a mean of 16 months. Mortality and the incidence of coronary events were reduced significantly and the effect was particularly noticeable in patients without overt heart failure.

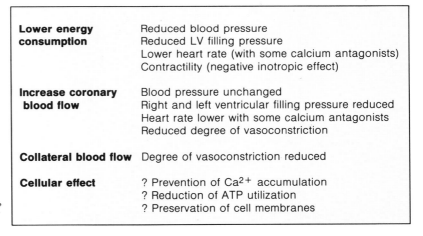

Lower energy consumption	Reduced blood pressure Reduced LV filling pressure Lower heart rate (with some calcium antagonists) Contractility (negative inotropic effect)
Increase coronary blood flow	Blood pressure unchanged Right and left ventricular filling pressure reduced Heart rate lower with some calcium antagonists Reduced degree of vasoconstriction
Collateral blood flow	Degree of vasoconstriction reduced
Cellular effect	? Prevention of Ca^{2+} accumulation ? Reduction of ATP utilization ? Preservation of cell membranes

Fig. 11. Reasons for 'protection' of the myocardium.

One explanation for these contrasting results is that the hazardous effects of calcium antagonists (negative inotropic effect, early hypotensive effect, reflex tachycardia, early activation of the sympathetic and renin–angiotensin systems) dominate in the presence of heart failure whereas the advantage is seen in other patients. A further consideration is that the formulation of drugs used in the many trials of calcium antagonists in myocardial infarction had a short duration of action and would have induced an early fall in blood pressure. Newer formulations and newer drugs may have different effects in ischaemia.

Calcium antagonists in heart failure

Because calcium antagonists had been shown to be advantageous in animal experiments and had properties such as vasodilatation which were anticipated to be of benefit, they have been investigated in heart failure. Initial results for acute haemodynamics were

Study	Year	Drug	Patients	Duration	CK-MB	Reinfarction	Mortality
Myocardial infarction							
Muller *et al*	1984	Nifedipine	171	6 months	0	0	0
Bussman *et al*	1984	Verapamil	54	48 hours	30%	–	–
Gottlieb *et al*	1984	Nifedipine	132	6 weeks	0	0	0
Norwegian	1984	Nifedipine	227	6 weeks	–	0	0
Danish Study	1984	Verapamil	1436	12 months	0	–	0
SPRINT	1986	Nifedipine	2279	12 months	–	0	0
TRENT	1986	Nifedipine	4491	1 month	–	–	0
MDPIT	1986	Diltiazem	576	14 days	–	$P < 0.06$	–
MDPIT	1988	Diltiazem	2466	25 months	–	0	0
DAVIT II	1990	Verapamil	1775	16 months	–	$P < 0.07$	$P < 0.05$
Unstable angina							
Muller *et al*	1984	Nifedipine	126	–	–	–	0
HINT	1986	Nifedipine	515	–	–	–	0

Fig. 12. Calcium antagonists in acute myocardial infarction and unstable angina.

Fig. 13. Mortality trials in acute myocardial infarction. Adapted by permission (Yusuf *et al. Cardiovasc Drugs Ther* 1987; **1**: 343–344).

	Drug	Trials	Deaths	
			Control	Drug
Short-term trials	Diltiazem	1	11/287	9/289
	Nifedipine	5	198/2594	175/2600
	Verapamil	1	0/8	2/9
Long-term trials	Diltiazem	1	167/1234	166/1232
	Nifedipine	1	66/1140	64/1139
	Lidoflazine	1	177/896	168/896
	Verapamil	1	109/717	118/719
	Total	11	728/6876 (11%)	702/6884 (10%)

	No. of trials	No. of patients	% Reduction of	
			Mortality	Infarction
Beta blockers	25	23000	−22*	−27*
Antiplatelet drugs	10	18500	−11*	−31*
Calcium antagonists	4	9000	+6	–
Cholesterol reduction	22	40000	−10*	−17*
Blood pressure Rx	9	43000	−11*	− 8*
Exercise	9	4300	−19*	+3
* $P < 0.05$				

Fig. 14. Secondary reduction of mortality and further infarction: meta-analysis of long-term trials. Data from Yusuf *et al. JAMA* 1988; **260**:2088–2093 and 2259–2263.

encouraging but, when the drugs were tested over the long term, deterioration of the patient was commonly observed [15,16]. This was related to the negative inotropic action of calcium antagonists but may have also been the consequence of activation of the sympathetic nervous system and the renin–angiotensin system. A recent prospective, randomized, double-blind trial of nifedipine compared with nitrates in 28 patients showed a deterioration with the calcium antagonist [16]. Only two trials comparing calcium antagonists with placebo in heart failure fulfil reasonable criteria for a double-blind, randomized trial. In one [39], felodipine was shown in 15 patients not to increase exercise time or improve symptoms, and caused fluid retention despite an increase in cardiac output. In the second [40], amlodipine was reported in 118 patients to improve exercise capacity and symptoms.

Trial	Size	Years	CHD death		Total death		% Reduction		Lives saved/ 1000 treated
			Int.	Plac.	Int.	Plac.	CHD	Total	
Multiple interventions									
WHO	60881	6	428	450	1325	1341	5	1	0.5
Goteborg	30000	12	462	461	1293	1318	0	1.9	1.7
MRFIT	12866	7	115	124	265	260	7	+2	+0.8
Helsinki	1222	5	4	4	10	5	0	+50	+8
Oslo	1232	5	6	13	16	23	54	30	11
Cholesterol									
WHO (clof.)	15745	5	54	48	162	127	+13	+28	+4
LRC-CPPT	3806	7	32	44	68	71	27	4	1.6
Gemfibrozil	4081	5	6	8	45	42	25	+7	+1.5
Smoking									
Whitehall	1445	10	49	62	123	128	21	4	7
Hypertension									
8 trials	17314	–	–	–	784	887	–	12	12
MRC	17354	5	106	97	248	253	+9	2	0.6

Fig. 15. Interventional trials in coronary heart disease. Data from McCormick and Skrabanek, *Lancet* 1988; **ii**:839.

Evidence for the reversal of atheroma in man

Before considering the evidence that calcium antagonists can influence the development of atheroma, it is appropriate to consider the evidence that any intervention can be shown to do that in man. Regression of both coronary and aortic atheroma has been shown in animal models. Most studies in man have used diet or drug therapy to lower blood cholesterol. Early studies of drug intervention were undertaken on the femoral arteries, but several studies have now been reported on progression of atheroma in coronary arteries.

The Leiden Intervention Trial [41] was a prospective trial of a vegetarian diet, low in cholesterol, and with a polyunsaturated to saturated fat ratio of greater than 2. Repeat angiography took place at years in 39 patients. The total blood cholesterol was 7.0 mmol/litre (271 mg/dl). No progression was observed in 18 patients (46%) and progression was associated with the severity of the blood lipid abnormality. There was no control group.

Kuo *et al.* [42] reported on 25 patients with type II hyperlipoproteinaemia who were treated for 7$\frac{1}{2}$ years with diet and colestipol. The mean total blood cholesterol was 11.3 mmol/litre. Repeat coronary angiograms in 12 patients revealed no difference in the size of lesions in eight and variable progression in four. There was no control group of patients. Nash *et al.* [43] studied the effects of colestipol in 36 patients with an average total cholesterol of 6.5 mmol/litre over 23 months. The cholesterol level was reduced by 21% and disease progressed in 17%. This was compared with 48% in the 'controls'. The study was not randomized or controlled. Nikkila *et al.* [44] treated 28 patients with clofibrate and/or nicotinic acid for 7 years. Blood cholesterol was 7.2 mmol/litre and fell by 18%. Progression occurred in 16%, compared with 32% in the 'controls'. Again, the controls were not randomized. The best early trial was organized by the National Heart, Lung and Blood Institute in the United States (NHLBI study) [45]. This was a randomized, placebo-controlled study on 59 patients receiving cholestyramine and 57 patients receiving placebo over a period of 5 years. The total blood cholesterol level was reduced by 17% in the treated group and increased by 1% in the control group. Disease progression occurred in 32% of patients and 49% of controls, the difference being not significant. The angiograms were assessed visually. It was suggested that the progression of disease was reduced in those with severe disease at the time of admission to the study.

More recently, the Cholesterol Lowering Atherosclerosis Study (CLAS) [46] reported the effects of colestipol and niacin in high doses given for 2 years to 80 patients. A comparison with 82 patients on placebo was made by visual analysis of the angiogram. The total blood cholesterol was reduced by 26 and 4% in the two groups ($P < 0.002$). The angiogram were assessed by a panel of experts visually. Regression occurred in 16% of patients on active treatment and in only 2% on placebo. The figures for progression were 39%, compared with 61% ($P < 0.03$). Regression occurred in 16.2 treated patients compared with 2.4% in the placebo group ($P < 0.002$). These findings were accompanied by evidence of clinical benefit. An important point about this trial is that the patients had a total blood cholesterol level at the start of the trial of only 6.4 mmol/litre. The benefit was shown in patients regardless of the initial cholesterol level. The treatment was aggressive and side effects were common.

The most recent clinical study is the Familial Atherosclerosis Treatment Study (FATS) [47]. This was a placebo-controlled, randomized study. One hundred and forty-six patients were randomized to placebo, lovastatin and colestipol, or niacin and colestipol. All patients received dietary advice. The angiograms were analysed by computer methods after $2\frac{1}{2}$ years. The mean total blood cholesterol level at entry was 7.0 mmol/litre. Cholesterol was reduced by more than 30% in all the treated groups. In the placebo group progression was observed in 46% and regression in 11%. In the treated groups progression occurred in 21 and 25%, and regression in 32 and 39%, respectively ($P < 0.005$). The reduction of atheroma was accompanied by indications of clinical benefit.

A third trial tested not the effects of a drug but of partial ileal bypass surgery [48]. In this trial, 838 patients were randomized to either surgery or a control group. The mean follow-up time was 9.7 years. The mean cholesterol level fell from 6.1 to 4.7 mmol/litre. Total mortality and that attributed to coronary artery disease were unaltered. Overall mortality was reduced in a subgroup with an ejection fraction greater than 50%. Combined endpoints did show a significant reduction and the number of patients undergoing cardiac surgery was less in the operated group. Repeat coronary angiograms were performed in a large proportion of the patients in the trial. The severity of atheroma in the coronary arteries was reduced by the intervention ($P < 0.002$) but the proportion of patients with positive exercise tests was unchanged.

Thus, the three most recent and best designed studies have been able to demonstrate a reduction in the progression of atheroma. Two of the trials have also provided evidence of regression of atheroma as a result of therapeutic intervention aimed at the reduction of blood cholesterol.

Clinical evidence for reversal of atheroma by calcium antagonists

Two randomized, placebo-controlled studies [13,14] have reported on the effects of calcium antagonists on atheroma in the coronary arteries. Both studies were started after the availability of animal evidence that regression could result from long-term treatment with a calcium antagonist [22,23].

The first study was the International Nifedipine Trial on Antiatherosclerotic Therapy (INTACT), coordinated in Germany and the Netherlands [13,49]. No less than 425 patients were enrolled and randomized to treatment with nifedipine 20 mg four times a day or placebo. A second angiogram was performed after 3 years and both were subjected to sophisticated computer analysis. The mean total cholesterol level at entry was 6.75 mmol/litre. The primary purpose of this study was to show regression or at least lack of progression of coronary lesions in patients treated with nifedipine. In this respect the study was negative in that no impact on established lesions was shown (Fig. 16). A secondary aim was to assess the frequency of the appearance of new lesions. There was a 28% reduction in the number of new lesions per patient ($P < 0.03$). The appearance of a new lesion was defined as a lesion reducing the diameter by 20% or more. In the trial there were 12 deaths (eight cardiac) in the nifedipine group and two (both cardiac deaths) in the placebo group. This difference did reach significance for total deaths but not for cardiac deaths. This result is very likely to have occurred by chance. Only five of the deaths were in patients taking the drug at the time of death.

In the second study, by Waters *et al.* in Canada [14], 383 patients were randomized to treatment with nicardipine 30 mg three times a day or placebo. Coronary angiography was repeated after 2 years and the angiograms were analysed by a computer technique. The baseline total blood cholesterol level was 6.74 mmol/litre. The findings were essentially identical to those reported in the INTACT study. No difference in the regression or progression of established coronary lesions could be shown between the treated and placebo

Study	Drug	No. in located group	Progression		Regression		No change	
			Drug	Control	Drug	Control	Drug	Control
Loaldi et al. (1989)	Nifedipine	39	31%	53%	18%	8%	51%	39%
INTACT (1990)	Nifedipine	173	23%	24%	10%	14%	62%	64%
Waters et al. (1990)	Nicardipine	192	9%	10.5%	3.7%	3.3%	87.3%	87.2%
Gottlieb et al. (1989)	Nifedipine	72	33%	48%	–	–	–	–

Fig. 16. Summary of trial to assess the effect of calcium antagonists on coronary atheroma in man.

groups. However, there was a reduction in the progression of small or new lesions from 27 to 15% ($P<0.046$).

Two further studies are relevant. Gottlieb et al. [50] have reported in an abstract that nifedipine started early after coronary bypass surgery reduced the size of lesions in vein grafts over a period of one year. Loaldi et al. [51] repeated coronary angiography after 2 years in 39 patients on nifedipine (20 mg four times a day), 36 on propranolol (80 mg four times a day), and 38 on isosorbide dinitrate (40 mg two times daily). The patients were not randomly assigned to treatment and the investigation was not blind or placebo controlled. The progression of old and new lesions was significantly reduced ($P<0.05$). Regression occurred in only 13 but was more common in those taking nifedipine ($P<0.05$). The two large studies studies were randomized, placebo-controlled and carefully done. The conclusion was rather unexpected but was the same in both, namely that there was a reduction in the appearance of new lesions. This finding is in accord with the short-term animal experiments and has clear clinical significance. It might be argued that regression or lack of progression in the size of an atheromatous plaque could not be expected to be demonstrated in an advanced lesion because of the extent of fibrosis and calcification which may be present. If, however, that argument were true then the NHLBI [45], CLAS [46], FATS [47] and Program on the Surgical Control of the Hyperlipidemias (POSCH) [48] studies should not have been able to show an effect as a result of therapy directed at impairing lipid metabolism. It may be that some as yet unidentified biological process in the early development of atheromatous lesions is sensitive to calcium antagonists. If that is shown to be true, then the calcium antagonists would have a rather special role in the treatment of coronary atherosclerosis.

Several mechanisms have been put forward to account for the effect of calcium antagonists on atheroma in animal experiments (Fig. 3). One possibility is that these results could be the consequence of haemodynamic or anti-ischaemic effects of the calcium antagonists. In the presence of the calcium antagonist, minor episodes of ischaemia may be less common. By causing physical or functional damage to the endothelium such episodes could contribute to the progression of atheromatous disease. Waters et al. [14] put forward an alternative argument: they suggested that the effect was due to the reduction of blood pressure. In support of that argument they showed a correlation between the fall in blood pressure and the reduction in the occurrence of new lesions. In the INTACT study [49] blood pressure was not reduced in those who were normotensive but was greatly reduced in those who had high blood pressures at the start of the study. However, a fall in blood pressure did not reduce the occurrence of myocardial infarction in a large number of controlled trials. Calcium antagonists do not in general reduce the blood pressure in those who are normotensive. Furthermore, in the study of Loaldi *et al.* [51], the benefit of calcium antagonists was shown despite treatments which lower the blood pressure equally.

Future prospects: impact of calcium antagonists on the therapeutic approach to ischaemic heart disease and hypertension

The calcium antagonists were originally introduced into clinical practice for the treatment of angina pectoris. Later they were used to treat hypertension. Large numbers of patients with these conditions are treated with calcium antagonists throughout the world. This group of drugs does not seem to be of benefit to all patients with acute myocardial infarction, unstable angina, or heart failure. Some patients with myocardial infarction do benefit, however, and it may be that subgroups of patients with heart failure, those with diastolic heart failure for example, may also be treated with advantage. The future use of these drugs, and others, in these conditions will depend on the identification of subsets of patients who are identifiable by simple clinical criteria and who can be shown to benefit. The new formulations of the calcium antagonists may bring real advantages.

That these drugs delay the development of new atherosclerotic lesions is an important additional feature. Whether this will ever be shown to affect the clinical manifestations of coronary artery disease is doubtful in view of the difficulties and size of such studies. A more useful approach is the study of the effect of these drugs on carefully selected groups of patients.

Preventive measures, correction of lipid abnormalities, and aspirin to modify platelet function are common and usual treatments for patients with atheromatous coronary artery disease. The evidence showing that calcium antagonists prevent the development of new lesions in the coronary arteries provides a new and novel reason for using them in the treatment of patients with coronary artery disease and hypertension. The latter is a major risk factor in the atherogenic process (as shown in the INTACT study with nifedipine [13]). The antiatherosclerotic effect of calcium antagonists could be of benefit to patients with hypertension or known coronary artery disease by preventing the enlargement of early lesions.

References

1. Simons LA: Interrelations of lipids and lipoproteins with coronary artery disease mortality in 19 countries. *Am J Cardiol* 1986; **57**:5G–10G.

2. GISSI Study: Effectiveness of intravenous thrombolytic treatment in acute myocardial infarction. *Lancet* 1986; i:397–401.
3. ISIS-2 (Second International Study of Infarct Survival) Collaborative

Group: Randomized trial of intravenous streptokinase, oral aspirin, both or neither among 17,189 cases of suspected acute myocardial infarction: ISIS-2. *Lancet* 1988; ii:349–360.

4. Stehbens WE: An appraisal of the epidemic rise of coronary heart disease and its decline. *Lancet* 1987; i:606–610.

5. Corday E, Ryden L: Why some physicians have concerns about the cholesterol awareness program. *J Am Coll Cardiol* 1989; **13**:497–502.

6. Oliver MF: Prevention of coronary heart disease – propaganda, promises, problems, and prospects. *Circulation* 1986; **73**:1–9.

7. Brett AS: Treating hypercholesterolaemia: how should practicing physicians interpret the published data from patients? *N Engl J Med* 1989; **321**:676–680.

8. Leaf A: Management of hypercholesterolemia: are preventative interventions advisable? *N Engl J Med* 1989; **321**:680–684.

9. The NIH Consensus Development Conference to Lower Blood Cholesterol for Prevention of Heart Disease. *JAMA* 1985; **253**:2080–2086.

10. Study Group, European Atherosclerosis Society: Strategies for the prevention of coronary heart disease: a policy statement of the European Atherosclerosis Society. *Eur Heart J* 1987; **8**:77–88.

11. The British Cardiac Society Working Party on Coronary Prevention: conclusions and recommendations. *Br Heart J* 1987; **57**:188–189.

12. Holme I: An analysis of randomized trials evaluating the effect of cholesterol reduction on total mortality and coronary heart disease incidence *Circulation* 1990; **82**:1916–1924.

13. Lichtlen PR, Hugenholtz PG, Rafflenbeul W, Hecker H, Jost S, Deckers JW: Retardation of angiographic progression of coronary artery disease by nifedipine. Results of the International Nifedipine Trial on Antiatherosclerotic Therapy (INTACT). *Lancet* 1990; **335**: 1109–1113.

14. Waters D *et al.*: A Controlled clinical trial to assess the effect of a calcium channel blocker on the progression of coronary atherosclerosis. *Circulation* 1990; **82**:1940–1953.

15. Packer M: Calcium channel blockers in chronic heart failure. *Circulation* 1990; **82**:2254–2257.

16. Elkayam U, Weber L, McKay C, Rahimtoola S: Spectrum of acute hemodynamic effects of nifedipine in severe chronic congestive heart failure. *Am J Cardiol* 1985; **56**:560–566.

17. Yusuf *et al.*: Meta-analysis. *JAMA* 1988; **260**:2088–2093 and 2259–2263.

18. Held PH, Yusuf, Furberg CD: Calcium channel blockers in acute myocardial infarction and unstable angina: an overview. *Br Med J* 1989; **299**:1187–1192.

19. The Multicentre Diltiazem Postinfarction Trial Research Group: The effect of diltiazem on mortality and reinfarction after myocardial infarction. *N Engl J Med* 1988; **319**:385–392.

20. The Multicentre Diltiazem Postinfarction Research Group: Diltiazem increases late-onset congestive heart failure in post-infarction patients with early reduction in ejection fraction. *Circulation* 1991; **83**:52–60.

21. The Danish Study Group on Verapamil in Myocardial Infarction: Effect of verapamil on mortality and major events after acute myocardial infarction (The Danish Verapamil Infarction Trial II – DAVIT II). *Am J Cardiol* 1990; **66**:779–785.

22. Fleckenstein A, Fleckenstein-Grün G: Cardiovascular protection by calcium Ca^{2+} antagonist. *Eur Heart J* 1980; (suppl B):15–21.

23. Henry PD: Calcium antagonists as antiatherogenic agents. *Ann NY Acad Sci* 1988; **522**:411–419.

24. Barker DJP: The intrauterine origins of cardiovascular and obstructive lung disease in adult life. *J R Coll Phys* 1991; **25**:129–133.

25. Davies MJ, Thomas AC: Plaque fissuring – the cause of acute myocardial infarction, sudden ischemic death, and crescendo angina. *Br Heart J* 1985; **53**: 363–373.

26. Falk E: Plaque rupture with severe pre-existing stenosis precipitating coronary thrombosis. Characteristics of coronary atherosclerosis plaques underlying fatal occlusive thrombi. *Br Heart J* 1983; **50**: 127–134.

27. Richardson PD, Davies MJ, Born GVR: Influence of plaque configuration and stress distribution on fissuring of coronary atherosclerotic plaques. *Lancet* 1989; ii: 941–944.

28. Meade TW *et al.*: Haemostatic function and ischaemic heart disease: Principal results of the Northwick Park Heart Study. *Lancet* 1986; ii:533–538.

29. Moore TJ: The cholesterol myth. *The Atlantic Monthly*. September 1989.

30. Hawkes N: Leave us to our chips: this hectoring is even worse. *The Times*. 22 September 1990.

31. McCormick J, Skrabanek P: Coronary heart disease is not preventable by population interventions. *Lancet* 1988; ii: 839–841.

32. Leitch D: Who should have their cholesterol concentration measured? What experts in the United Kingdom suggest. *Br Med J* 1989; **298**:1615–1616.

33. Anderson KM, Castelli WP, Levy D: Cholesterol and mortality. 30 years of follow-up from the Framingham Study. *JAMA* 1987; **257**:2176–2180.

34. Rossouw JE: The value of lowering cholesterol after myocardial infarction. *N Engl J Med* 1990; **323**:1112–1119.

35. Muldoon MF, Manuck SB, Matthews KA: Lowering cholesterol concentrations and mortality: a quantitative review of primary prevention trials. *Br Med J* 1990; **301**:309–314.

36. Isles CG, Hole DJ, Hawthorne VM, Lever AF: Plasma cholesterol, coronary heart disease and cancer in the Renfrew and Paisley survey. *Br Med J* 1989; **298**: 920–924.

37. Editorial: Low cholesterol and increased risk. *Lancet* 1989; ii:1423–1425.

38. Opie LH: Reperfusion injury and calcium-antagonists. *Cardiologia* 1990; **35**(suppl 1 al n 12):213–221.

39. Tan LB, Murray RG, Littler WA: Felodipine in patients with chronic congestive heart failure: discrepant haemodynamic and clinical effects. *Br Heart J* 1987; **58**:122–128.

40. Packer M *et al.*: Randomized, multicentre, double-blind, placebo-controlled evaluation of amlodipine in patients with mild to moderate heart failure. *J Am Coll Cardiol* 1991; **17**:274A.

41. Arntzenius AC, Kromnout D, Barth JD: Diet, lipoproteins and the progression of coronary atherosclerosis. The Leiden intervention trial. *N Engl J Med* 1985; **312**:805–811.

42. Kuo PT, Hayase K, Koskis JB, Moreyra AE: Use of combined diet and colestipol in long-term (7–7$\frac{1}{2}$ years) treatment of patients with type II hyperlipoproteinaemia. *Circulation* 1979; **59**:199–211.

43. Nash DT, Gensini G, Esente P: The progression of coronary atherosclerosis. *J Cardiac Rehab* 1984; **4**:21–26.

44. Nikkila EA, Viikinkoski P, Valle M, Frick MH: Prevention of progression of coronary atherosclerosis by treatment of hyperlipidaemia: a seven year prospective angiographic study. *Br Med J* 1984; **289**: 220–223.

45. Brensike JF, Levy RI, Kelsey SF *et al.*: Effects of therapy with cholestyramine on progression of coronary arteriosclerosis: results of the NHLBI Type II Coronary Intervention Study. *Circulation* 1984; **69**: 313–324.

46. Blankenhorn DH, Nessim SA, Johnson RL, Sanmarco ME, Azen SP, Caschen-Hemphill L: Beneficial effects of combined colestipol-niacin therapy on coronary atherosclerosis and coronary venous bypass grafts. *JAMA* 1987; **257**:3233–3240.

47. Brown G: Regression of coronary artery disease as a result of intensive lipid-lowering therapy in men with high levels of apolipoprotein B. *N Engl J Med* 1990; **323**:1289–1298.

48. Bughwald H: Effect of partial ileal bypass surgery on mortality and morbidity from coronary heart disease in patients with hypercholesterolemia. Report of the Program on the Surgical Control of the Hyperlipidemias (POSCH). *N Engl J Med* 1990; **323**:946–955.

49. Lichtlen PR *et al.*: Retardation of coronary artery disease in humans by the calcium-channel blocker nifedipine: results of the INTACT Study (International Nifedipine Trial on Antiatherosclerotic Therapy). *Cardiovasc Drugs Ther* 1990; **4**:1047–1068.

50. Gottlieb O *et al.*: Effect of nifedipine on the development of coronary bypass graft stenoses in high-risk patients: a randomized, double-blind, placebo-controlled trial. *Circulation* 1989; **80** (suppl II) [abstract].

51. Loaldi A, Polese A, Montorsi P, *et al.*: Comparison of nifedipine, propranolol and isosorbide dinitrate on angiographic progression and regression of coronary arterial narrowings in angina pectoris. *Am J Cardiol* 1989; **64**:433–439.

Index

Page numbers in *italics* indicate figures.